MW01030538

MORE PRAISE FOR

Raging Currents

Raging Currents is a powerful, important book. It's a "must read" not only for families and people struggling with these issues but also for health professionals, mental health workers, and all who care about mental health issues in our society. Dr. Davis offers how-to-strategies for navigating the health care system and coping with two mentally ill loved ones, as well as criticisms of our current mental health programs.

Lynne Masland, Ph.D.
A Century of Challenge and Change: Whatcom
Women and the YWCA

In *Raging Currents,* Nanette Davis has gifted us with candid and loving insight into the challenges of caring for a severely mentally-ill sister and son, while holding a family with five other children together, and working full time. She models courage and strength and delivers a realistic picture.

Skye Burn
Skye Burn Productions LLC

In this personal memoir, *Raging Currents,* Nanette Davis writes in intimate detail about her personal odyssey as caregiver for two loved ones: Sharon, who "lived a life tormented by self-loss," and a son, struggling to develop an identity. In this candid narrative, we experience Nanette's perseverance over many years in seeking help and providing care for her sister's schizophrenia and son's bipolar disease, despite family denial and the lack of support from the mental healthcare system. This story is a gift to anyone living with or knowing someone suffering from mental illness, impressing us on how love and persistence conquer all.

Nancy Canyon
Author of *Struck, Saltwater, and Dark Forest*

Raging Currents

Mental Illness and Family

A Memoir

Nanette J. Davis, Ph.D.

Raging Currents

Mental Illness and Family

Nanette J. Davis, Ph.D.

ISBN (Print Edition): 978-1-66788-251-2

ISBN (eBook Edition): 978-1-66788-252-9

© 2022. All rights reserved. No part of this publication
may be reproduced, distributed, or transmitted in any form
or by any means, including photocopying, recording, or
other electronic or mechanical methods, without the prior
written permission of the publisher, except in the case of
brief quotations embodied in critical reviews and certain
other noncommercial uses permitted by copyright law.

To My Beloved Family, all five generations, who are the wellspring of my inspiration and the love of my life.

Acknowledgments

Writing this memoir over nine years requires recognizing a host of steady supporters and patient readers. Most family members have heard portions of the story and provided feedback. My daughter, Katherine Delaney, offered a host of changes and commentaries on the family narrative. Alana-Christina Dittrich labored through the final version.

The book's most creative and critically acute readers have been my Western Washington University Retirement Association writers' group, including Evelyn Wright, Lynne Masland, Iris Jones, Suzanne Krogh, Troy Faith Ward, and Patricia Clark. I am deeply grateful for their careful listening and ongoing feedback on every chapter over countless years to complete this final long writing project of my life.

Nancy Canyon's inspiring classes helped to articulate sorrowful memories that cried out for expression.

I salute the late Ham Hayes, whose photographic expertise clarified the older photos and prepared all images for printing.

Richard Rohr, writer, mystic, and wisdom teacher, offered the profound metaphor for growing up in an alcoholic family I adopted for my book: "breathing underwater."

A heartfelt thanks to Lynda Jensen, editor extraordinaire, who poured through two different book versions before we settled on the one before you.

For Burl Harmon, creative chef, loving confidant, and stalwart supporter, I feel deep gratitude for your incredible fortitude in sharing difficult periods of my life and those of family members.

"*Until we have seen someone's darkness, we don't really know who that person is. Until we have forgiven someone's darkness, we really don't know what love is.*"

Marianne Williamson, *Illuminata*

Table of Contents

Part Three

Breathing Underwater

It happened without warning. One late spring, Uncle Fred and my father agreed to teach us to swim. The day was perfect. Mid-June, the blue sky swooped down to embrace us while the tender breeze softened the sun's intense heat. The other girls were giddy, waiting for this afternoon of frolicking. Secretly, I was terrified of the water and wanted to get this ordeal over with.

The river, a tributary of the grand Illinois, has a rapidly churning current, a dangerously deep depth, and a muddy shore that sucks small feet into its squishy surface. We barely arrived at the water's edge when Daddy abruptly grabbed me, lifting my entire body over his head straight into the brink. Whoosh! Splat! These were the sounds of my nine-year-old self being thrown into the river by my trickster father.

A non-swimmer aiming to overcome the initial shock of icy water must learn to flail arms while kicking ferociously to reach the shore, surviving by rapid responses to trial and error and unconscious actions engaged for survival. Some manage it; others don't. My dear lost sister, Sharon, never mastered the drowning waters of our addicted family.

A mother's alcoholism, a father's denial. Sharon must have been caught in the current of opposing realities, tormenting her sensitive psyche. Was she the proverbial canary in the coal mine, warning us of dangers? Were my flailing reactions supportive, or did they drag us both down?

2 · NANETTE J. DAVIS, PH.D.

Dog paddling my way across the vicious current that fateful day, I managed to get to safe ground. Shortly after my near disaster, Sharon swept away, slipped helplessly into the muddy waters. Rescued, yes. Alive, yes. Still, the image of her sinking and going under remains a powerful simile of Sharon's life's journey.

The swimming lessons describe more than Sharon and me and how the same river washed over us differently. My son, Michael, caught in the strong currents of social disorder in the 1970s, began a long journey with mental illness in his teens. Mike was rescued, with early intervention pulling him out of one psychotic episode after another. My son never completely drowned because my family—mainly my late husband, Jim, myself, and to a lesser extent, Mike's siblings—refused to allow him to get over his head. Despite his resistance and relapses pulling us down, we held on tight to our drowning boy. All of us rescuers fell prey to the burden of care and abuse, some with lifelong consequences.

The story of a mother's alcoholism, a sister's schizophrenia, and a son's bipolar disease points to a genetic connection. But the social triggers and protective factors swamping my sister and my son show sharp differences. Sadly, their struggles to live with the psychiatric disruptions appear similar at some level. At another level, Mike has complicated his life with alcohol and drugs that trigger severe symptoms when taken to excess. His life can only be described as one in shambles during these episodes.

As a caregiver for two loved ones, I often felt as lost as they were. Neither my loved ones nor I have been fully released from the raging currents of the disease. I wrestled with Sharon's mental illness until her death, believing I could somehow cure her. Sharon managed to have a peaceful oasis at the end of her life but never escaped the illness. Michael continues to have challenges and relapses that afflict him physically and mentally. But when he is hospitalized and supervised by the mental health system, he returns to a normal life. Unfortunately, his relapses often prevent him from seeking relief.

This memoir, based on conversations, journals, documents, interviews, close observation, and experience, ultimately depends on the author's perspective and memory. Both can be flawed instruments. A mother's perception of her child's mental illness differs sharply from a sister's perspective. Despite taking responsibility, I knew it was never my fault when Sharon desdended into madness.

The opposite was the case with my son, for whom I shared that concern with my husband. I still struggle with the Twelve-Step recommendation: let go and let God. But I know that loving detachment means that we continue to love our mentally ill child or other loved one while allowing them to make their own choices, however grim, and to pursue their own journey.

Memory has more weaknesses than a biased perspective for writing a convincing story. I join the ranks of those writers who know that their narratives are unlikely to be shared and may even be denied by family members. We all live separate lives, with memories unique to each. For instance, my mother regaled me, as the oldest child in the family, with endless accounts of her parents and her childhood, her early marriage years, and her disappointments and griefs. I believe I am the sole recipient of those chronicles.

The most sketchy evidence is Sharon's lost years on her own and unavailable to me. Those years had to be filled in by conversations with institutional staff, official documents provided for legal guardians, and general observations of patients and their routines.

I took the liberty of changing some names for the privacy of the parties.

Finally, I hope my research skills, formerly applied to sociological matters, are reflected in this effort to write my story as truthfully and accurately as possible.

These are our stories. I cared for a sister who languished in the dark recesses of mental illness for almost all of her adult life. I cared for a son who, from time to time, escaped the worst of the raging currents. None of us emerged unscarred.

Part One

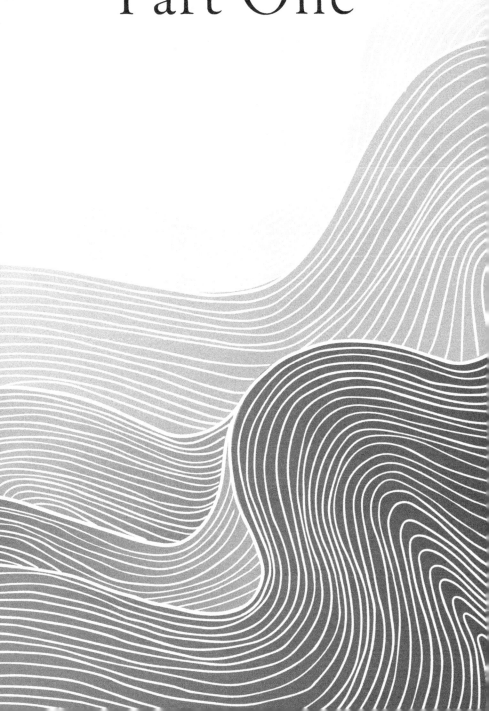

CHAPTER ONE

Born into Turmoil

I n 1936, our family lived in North Chicago, home to a polyglot of peoples: Catholic, Protestant, and Jewish religions; German, Irish, Russian, Italian, and Polish nationalities. Blocks of apartment buildings produced colliding cultures and a surplus of outdoor-bound youngsters, whose play areas remained confined to streets or concrete-filled backyards. The avenue contained not only our neighborhood children but other kids, who occasionally swarmed into our area from lower-income housing located a few blocks away, always ready for a fight. A kid had to be on the lookout every minute for danger. I doubt if our parents ever had a clue.

These Northside Chicago neighborhoods, abundant with children, carried their ethnically biased parents' fears and distrust of others. Adults sometimes encouraged an altercation, pushing their little ones into combat. Others used the children's verbal or physical collisions as an excuse for a run-in with a "kike," a "wop," a "polak," a "kraut," or a "mick," or any one of a despised ethnicity or religion other than those whose ancestors were born in England or Wales.

Because of our mixed household, comprised of my Irish Catholic mother, Alice, and my German Protestant father, Van—an ethnic mingling much derided by both groups—I became the frequent target of local youth. Aggressive kids sought to keep in line any hybrid form of human, even though most of those children hardly had pedigreed backgrounds.

I quickly picked up on the local conventions: attack first and retreat fast. I was the firstborn, a fierce little kid, the only girl ready to battle with every brat in the neighborhood. You could say I was looking for trouble.

I wanted to find a place in my family. I lived in Eden until sister Marilyn's arrival. Before she was born, I had an idyllic early childhood with both parents fixated on my infant accomplishments—walking, talking, solo eating—all exclaimed over. After baby sister number one's birth, I fell into the second rank. Jealousy aggravated my bowels, and constipation became a lifelong condition. Chronic irritation ignited my nerves resulting in a jumpiness and hyperactivity that plagued me for years.

I also wanted to find a place in this neighborhood. Lacking an older brother, I had to step forward, make a stand, and establish my authority in the neighborhood, at least among the small fry. On a grim winter day edging toward Christmas, I picked my target. I decided to go after 7-year-old Noah, a nearsighted, rickety boy, hardly my enemy, whose bowlegged limbs could never catch up with my cod-liver-oil-fed sturdy legs.

My parents prepared me for battle from infancy, spooning the dreadful slick syrup into my resistant mouth. Even though another baby sister was due to arrive home soon, it was the right day for me to move against my adversary. After all, nobody was around to stop me.

At age five, short for my age but admittedly a terror, I sized up my new birthday jump rope as a possible weapon. I estimated that the heavy piece of equipment would do a better job than my small fists at subduing smarty-pants Noah. I had cultivated my rope trick days before, twirling it like I'd seen my uncle Fred do when he wanted to catch a calf. Forget the rope. I'd hit him with the wooden handles. Then he'd know who the boss was and stay out of my way. I waited for the right moment.

I was ready when poor, stunted Noah came stumbling out of his third-floor walk-up that Friday afternoon.

To accomplish the deed, I deployed a surprise attack. Grasping the rope at its center, I swung the handles expertly as I walked up to my victim. He grinned at me, then grimaced and took a step back. I went after him and smashed the two handles into Noah's face, knocking off his glasses and leaving him stunned and disoriented. He collapsed into a heap, a bloody and battered undersized boy.

"That'll show you," I shouted as I began my terror-filled sprint to safety. After dashing through a dozen or so yards, slowed down by my frequent encounters with icy, billowing laundry, I felt sure Noah's pals would rat on me. I could be in hot water. Where to go? I made a dash for our apartment lobby to a small mail-room refuge, the perfect place to cower until things blew over.

I suppose I chose the wrong day, maybe even the wrong kid, for executing this braggadocio act. My parents, overwrought from my mother's long labor and delivery, planned to bring baby Sharon home from the hospital. Freezing winds off Lake Michigan that December 16th made the transition from Evanston Hospital to our Chicago north-side apartment a bone-chilling event. I heard the car pull into the alley, and curious, I left my perch to check out the new baby.

Dashing out to the backyard as Daddy pulled into the garage, I took one look at my mother hunched inside her coat, carrying a tiny bundle. I decided I did not want or need another sister at that moment. The creeping increase in children horrified me. One more bawling baby was one too many. I retreated and returned to my refuge, vowing to ignore this additional encumbrance Mommy insisted on bringing into our crowded apartment.

An hour later, Daddy discovered me huddled, face between my knees, blubbering in anguish. What have I done? As he leaned over, quietly lifting my face to meet his eyes, I learned, in a single moment, an essential truth: my father's expression signaled something was terribly wrong. I waited for his usual punishment to ease the tension: a firm spanking and mild body shaking to remember an auspicious transgression better. Instead, he spoke softly.

"Do you know Noah's parents are heartbroken about their son's injuries? He has to see a doctor. They're going to make me pay for the doctor and maybe even bring a lawsuit. His dad's a lawyer, you know."

Not his words, but the tone of his voice let me know this was the gravest moment of my life. No comment was made about either the new baby or my exhausted mother.

Rather than anger, Daddy expressed his concern for the child, the parents' misery, his deep-seated worry about money, and my unfortunate behavior. He resisted the idea (I would only understand later) of having to pay out all that money to a lawyer. A wise decision, he insisted, would be for me to make amends, not him.

With my paltry allowance of 10 cents a week, I paid this despised boy for damages incurred. Of course, my father paid the family the total damages.

My father's sensible approach won the day and avoided the dreaded legal suit. Noah survived with front teeth missing, a deep scar on his forehead, and an avowed desire to spend his free time in the public library. A few months later, I contracted scarlet fever and spent six weeks in a foul-smelling hospital isolation ward, seeing my weeping parents only through a window. I gagged and coughed my way through the life-threatening illness.

When I returned home, limp and tottering from the hospital, the jump rope incident had been nearly forgotten, although I continued my allowance payments until our family moved away. Mommy and Daddy were overwhelmingly grateful I did not die, unlike my country cousin, 12-year-old Amanda. Lacking a decent hospital and the new sulfa drugs, the scourge of scarlet fever demolished the most strenuous efforts of Aunt Cappa and Uncle Floyd to save their only surviving child.

Daddy wept bitter tears over his sister's loss of her child. Although pregnant twelve times, the couple saw eleven infants die before their 12-year-old daughter's death, all of them either stillborn or newborn. For those lucky few of us who survived the scourge of scarlet fever, we carry the memory of the streptococci deep within our cells, either with rheumatic fever or, in my case, a heart murmur.

Daddy, meanwhile, could not seem to recoup his losses from the stock market crash a few years earlier and continued to wring his hands over costs: monstrous medical bills—after all, families had no health insurance in the 1930s—household demands, and rising prices. I heard him often arguing with Mommy about her expenses, which in his mind were extravagant.

"Who needs lipstick, fancy shampoos, hair gloss, and face cream? And toothpaste? That's the last straw. That's an outrageous waste of time and money."

"Use soda for your teeth, like me," he insisted. "More healthy and cleansing." My mother, Alice, shuddered and bit her lip. She had no plans to change her expenditures, especially not to use plain soda, like poor people, to clean her sparkling white teeth. Daddy had already lost four teeth and was barely in his mid-thirties. He wasn't the right person to advise her about dental care.

I suspect my father's increasing harshness within the family and his high need for control date from this period. The apprehension hovering over the new middle class in the 1930s cannot be overstated. Chronic, unremitting, and impersonal, the foreboding presence of poverty never left him during those formative years while they raised three daughters.

As for baby Sharon, she had a problematic reception in her new family. Our parents were preoccupied with the possible loss of their firstborn child. I was ill and hospitalized for the first months of her life, while two-year-old Marilyn was bereft of loving care during my mother's last months of pregnancy. Daddy suffered financial headaches, and Mommy suffered household disorders even with our live-in, grossly inexperienced maid from Alabama. She was hardly the right fit for my father's demanding domestic order but tried her best to help Mommy recuperate from childbirth and care for two infants.

Sharon's arrival, forever linked to a time of family turbulence and anguish, had all the earmarks of just one more unbearable affliction an overburdened man must carry. Her haunted beginning may have pointed to Sharon's future difficulties growing up. Awkward, reticent, and too often withdrawn as a child, Sharon struggled in a household of intense energies and unresolved conflicts.

As for me, occasional parental leniencies, like trips to the family farm and solo visits to Grandma Anna in Chicago, helped defray the household tensions and made me feel quite special.

CHAPTER TWO

Neglect of A Beloved Grandmother

O n what must be the hottest August day ever, I received the exciting news about Mommy's mother. Not every 10-year-old girl had a chance to travel on her own to visit Grandma Anna Monaghan.

"Hi Grandma, Mommy and Daddy say I can stay with you for a whole week," I spouted excitedly over the phone, "and I don't have to take Marilyn or Sharon. They're too little to ride the "L" without Mommy or Daddy."

"That's wonderful, Sweetheart," she replied, her voice warm and smooth. "I'll see you on Saturday in time for our St. Theresa prayer circle. You shouldn't bring the other little girls, anyway. I don't have any space for them."

"Visiting Grandma—what a special experience," said Mommy after she hung up the phone for me. I agreed because I believed I was Grandma's favorite grandchild. I could be on my own—fearless, independent, eager to ride the Loop special.

The elevated train ride began in north Wilmette, then continued through Evanston before swooshing downward into the Chicago subway system and onward to Chicago's South side. At this point, the "L" was again elevated.

Grandma's street near Jackson Boulevard presented a busy thoroughfare where her Catholic Church, St. Teresa of the Little Flower, dominated the congested urban neighborhood.

After picking me up at the elevated station with its steep steps, Grandma offered me her small hand. I was nearly as tall as she, and we strolled ever so slowly to her apartment.

"Grandma has bad feet," Mommy warned me before I left home. "It's because she had so many children." Later I would learn that Grandma's feet hurt because she was old and worked too hard. Today, worn out after marching up and down the cliff-like transit steps to pick me up, Grandma dragged on my arm.

"Poor Grandma. She looks so frumpy, still wearing widow's weeds after all these years," Mommy would say, describing the black-on-black clothing that signaled Grandma's widow status. Even Grandma's shoes contributed to Mommy's complaints. The ugly and uncomfortable black lace-up shoes made my grandmother walk like a duck.

"I try to doll her up now and then," Mommy would say, "but Grandma will have none of it." Well-settled into widowhood, she shared her lot mainly with the other widowed rosary ladies who prayed every evening for the Monsignor's special intentions of the day.

* * *

"Now, Nanette, let me introduce you to my 'biys,'" Grandma said as she briskly began dinner preparations for ten. Grandma sure had a funny way of saying "boys." Mommy said it was because of Grandma's Irish background.

Grandma's "boys" were a mob of men ranging in age from 18 to well over 40, black hair slicked down, blue eyes staring out of sullen faces. All were unmarried, recent immigrants from Ireland, settling in Chicago with limited work skills and dashed dreams.

"There's Patrick, Johnny, Jimmy," recited Grandma, "Billy, Mike, Joe, Pete, and Ian."

All eight men usually bunked snugly into Grandma's three-bedroom, one-bath apartment. Grandma slept on a small cot in a tiny maid's room off the kitchen.

"Oh, Grandma, you have a lot of people staying here. Where'll we sleep?"

"We swap bedrooms. Mike and Johnny kindly offered up their room, so we can have the bigger bedroom and all the privacy we need while you're here."

"Why do you have so many 'biys'?"

"They haven't anyplace else to go, Honey. They're all alone in the world. I guess they're orphans. I like to help them out. But I tell them in no uncertain terms that demon alcohol won't pass their lips, not while they're with me—and they go to Mass every Sunday, without fail. No excuses."

I wouldn't learn until much later that Grandma would have been destitute without the room-and-board biys. I imagine that looking after a brood felt okay to her after raising seven of her own. Only one—the beautiful two-year-old, blond Eugene—lost when he picked up rotten food at the Illinois County Fair and died within two days of diarrhea-induced dehydration.

*　*　*

These men tell a different story than Grandma's flesh and blood, proudly third-generation American and very lace-curtain Irish. Anna was left bereft, struggling to make a living, often at her wit's end after Grandfather Monaghan died suddenly in his mid-fifties. Her surviving children—Betty, Marcella, Clarence, Paul, Alice, and Richard, once lived a comfortable life with their mother and father.

Her pride prevented her from asking for money from her grown, well-heeled offspring: Clarence, later renamed Patrick after he assumed the presidency of Packard Motor Car Company; Paul, who became an affluent insurance broker like his father; and Alice, who married well and became my mother, but didn't like her own mother very much. Betty and Marcella failed to secure financially prosperous husbands and remained impoverished sisters. Mommy loved her sisters and regularly sent discarded clothing and sometimes leftover perfume bottles to the pair, so they could "doll up."

Richard joined the Carmelite Order and became Father Pius—named after one of the many popes called Pius (we all, including Grandma, forget which one)—never had two coins to rub together to help his struggling mother. In fact, until World War II, Richard was a cloistered priest, locked into silence from age 13 by strict rules of obedience and rarely heard from. I suspect the war had a substantial impact on these shut-ins. One day, Fr. Pius arrived at our home on vacation, grinning happily. He showed off his officer's uniform and hugged Alice, his favorite sister, perhaps relieved that his confinement was over.

From that moment on, I became my uncle's greatest admirer. I loved mixing and serving his favorite cocktails every summer during my early adolescence, lighting his cigarettes, playing poker, and laughing at his jokes. During and after his military days, Fr. would arrive and remove all signs of clerical connection— the collar and black garments— then don one of the bright Hawaiian shirts my mother bought him and proceed to have a jolly good time. His favorite at-our-home activity happened to be singing with my mother, sometimes including the children; her nimble-fingered piano playing accompanied us all.

At some point, Mommy and her brother visited the out-of-town bars after Fr. taught himself to drive with Daddy's late model Buick. I remember Daddy being really angry sometimes when they came home late, accusing both of them of being "irresponsible brats" and receiving little more than giggles from the two miscreants.

During one of those summers Fr. Pius made the remarkable shift to Fr. Richard and to intimates, "Dick." The name change added another element to his transformation as a "hale-and-well-met fellow," according to my father. Though he and my mother only grudgingly visited Grandma, their reluctance opened the way for my nursing home visits during the last summer of her life. Jim, my fiancé, and I began filling in for her missing children. During my wedding engagement in the spring and summer of 1952, we routinely took trips out to Grandma Anna's Catholic nursing home, where we acted as stand-ins for Clarence and Alice; roles we played to the hilt.

*   *   *

Before Father Pius's transformation, though, when I was still ten and visiting Grandma on my own, dinner at Grandma's table was pretty much what my mother warned me: boiled beef and cabbage and undercooked potatoes, never mashed—no butter, no flavor, no complaints. The older men were more respectful, talkative, and at ease than the younger men. The men, heads down, carefully forked in their food, scraping their plates lightly, murmuring, "pass the salt, please," or "this is good, Mrs. Monaghan."

The meal finished, and the apple pie served on the same plate as the beef and potatoes, the men pushed their chairs back, stood, and carried their dishes from the dining room into the kitchen. Each dropped his burden, stacking plates in one pile, silverware in another, serving dishes to the side, and shuffled out of the kitchen into their assigned bedrooms. Once we finished washing and drying the enormous pile of dirty dishes, we left to attend the prayer circle at the church.

I loved the prayer circle. Grandma and all her friends, heads bowed, fingered their rosaries. While they murmured the sacred words, I took in the intoxicating scent of incense mixed with the aroma of the rich array of flowers surrounding the statue of beautiful St. Teresa. I could not keep my eyes open after my long "L" train ride, the excitement of coming to Chicago, and the biys staring at me while I nervously gulped down my food.

Could I go to hell never to be redeemed for dozing off? The piles of dirty dishes, plus Grandma's cross looks as long as the renters were around, had taken their toll.

"Wake up, girl," Grandma nudged. "You must pray along with us. God hates slackers, you know."

I sat up straighter and widened my sleepy eyes in an attempt to stay awake.

"I'll do better next time, Grandma," I whispered. "I promise."

She gave a heavy sigh, thumbing her rosary.

"Not sure you ever will, your Daddy not being Catholic. What is he, anyway? If I told Alice once, I told her a hundred times not to marry a non-Catholic."

"Not sure," I gulped, hating the conversation. "You're right, Grandma. I'd never marry a non-Catholic." I'd forget my promise soon enough, though.

Grandma refused to let go of the fact that my father did not have the Faith, and without faith, there was no hope for him, maybe for me too. I could see why my mother had such a hard time with her mother.

Trudging home, Grandma softened up a little.

"Now, Nanette, you pay attention, you hear me? Just say a prayer to our Lady, St. Teresa of the Little Flower. She'll grant your every wish." Before I could think of my wish, Grandma had a request for me. "Nanette, you have to promise me I'll never have to go to the Cook County Poorhouse." I assented eagerly to all of Grandma's promises.

"I promise, Grandma," I replied earnestly, even though I didn't have a shred of an idea of the whereabouts of the poor house. "But if you do have to go, I promise to go with you."

"Oh, no child, I have to go alone," she murmured, tears rolling down her cheeks, "just like the other old women of our parish without a penny to their names."

We returned to the silent living room, empty of radio and phonograph but reserved for just Grandma and me.

"You'll help me with the laundry for the mob tomorrow," said Grandma. "We'll start at dawn."

The following day, we hauled heavy jeans, underclothes, and work shirts to the basement and commenced washing one load after another in her old wringer washing machine. Once finished, we hung the soggy mass in the damp basement to dry. The prospect of a day devoted to dirty clothes in that dank basement still gives me the chills.

I managed to stay awake for subsequent church visits with Grandma, sometimes with her rosary friends, and sometimes just the two of us. I hated to admit that Grandma treated me as special because she thought she could save my soul against the evils of my father's faithless Protestant existence. My sisters never really knew Grandma as I did. They only saw her when she came to the house for Sunday afternoon dinner and sat demurely under our mother's unkind surveillance.

But I loved my Grandma Anna and wept silently, missing her once she deposited me after a long walk to the "L" station for my lonely, hour-long train trip home.

*　*　*

Once home, I told Daddy about my visit to Grandma, her biys, her sore feet, her ceiling-high stack of laundry, and her terror of going to the poor house, a fearsome destination in that epoch. Stricken, he turned to my mother.

"I told you we need to look into your mother's situation. I'll visit her next week after work. We may need to make some changes."

But Daddy didn't get there the following week nor for many weeks afterward, not until he received a call from a parish visitor, who said that Grandma lost herself in the neighborhood more than once and often went to the church for help. At that point, he took matters in hand.

Grandma didn't get banished to the Cook County Poorhouse or any house for that matter. Instead, her confused brain found refuge at a neighboring Catholic nursing home. There the nuns served as caregivers who alternated between tender mercies and harsh regimens. They fed and prayed over their charges, but they also required them to adhere to Lenten practices of fasting from meat and forcing them to kneel in church, regardless of the state of their old knees.

To this day, I'm not sure about the spiritual powers of St. Teresa of the Little Flower or my dear Grandma's efforts to turn me into a good Catholic. I know for sure that an angel touched me deeply that wonderful week when I was ten.

CHAPTER THREE

Near Misses

Sharon was a lost child, neglected by a preoccupied mother of two other daughters. Our father's life revolved around his daily trips to the Chicago office as an eager urban migrant in the 1930s, who, over time, moved from salesman to acting president of a cap and gown company. Daddy worked in one of the few industries that flourished during the Depression by allowing rentals of graduation apparel and choir robes for rich and poor alike. With Sharon's birth, though, he faced another disappointment: the wrong-gendered baby. She was just another girl.

When we were children, we often saw that little girl with dark, bobbed hair and wistful, blue eyes looking out the window or staring into space, her body rigid when reclining on her bed. Marilyn, my younger sister by three years and Sharon's older sister by two and one-half years, used the same bed for drying her expanding collection of artwork. I doubt Sharon had any space in that bedroom assigned for both children. I remember refusing to give her an inch in my private, wallpapered, and carpeted room. I held on to my privacy with tenacity without either parent considering the injustice of it all.

Sharon always seemed to be a sort of tag-along. When everyone stood ready for a trip or even seated in the car, someone would say: "Where's Sharon?"

"Oh boy, here we go again," I'd think as I took it upon myself to race upstairs and look for her.

"We're leaving, we're leaving," I'd call her. "Where are you?" Then I'd find her lying on the bed with a distant look.

We nearly lost her on one of our trips to Newton, in downstate Illinois, to visit the country relatives. We took long, winding trips from Wilmette through the northern Chicago suburbs, past Lake Zurich, where we spent one cold spring while the builders constructed our new house. Then we'd head straight south into farmland for hours past rolling fields of corn, oats, sorghum, alfalfa, and clover.

Usually, I claimed my seat next to the window, guarding my place as the older sister and official back door manager of the four-door Packard. Once, when I found Sharon upstairs, I lost my chance to put up my usual stink for first dibs. In a rush to get into the car, Sharon arrived last and commandeered my favorite spot. I found myself wedged between my two younger sisters. I must have been 9 or 10 years old as we hummed along the route to Grandma and Grandpa's house. I drove my sisters crazy by pinching their elbows and pushing them with chunky shoulders from one side to another. Suddenly, I became aware that Sharon wasn't pushing back at me anymore.

I turned toward four-year-old Sharon just in time to see her playing with the door handle. As I reached for her, the car door opened and swung out. Sharon held tightly to the handle, feet flying out into space, and our bodies swung momentarily out the door. In a moment that lasted forever, I grabbed a piece of her dress with one hand and her left leg with the other, awkwardly pulling her to safety.

Both parents began screaming—of course, at me.

"What have you done!" Daddy shouted, his right arm shooting out, ready to strike blows. "Are you insane, pushing your little sister out the door?" Mommy's eyes were angry slits as she stared at me.

"No, Daddy!" Marilyn shouted back, her blue eyes frantic. "Nanette pulled her back into the car. Didn't you see?" The voice of his trustworthy and ever-beloved daughter stayed his furious hand and rescued me.

Exonerated, I was briefly honored as heroic, becoming more significant than the "little helper" that day—my mother's favorite phrase. Instead, I became a savior, saint, and blessed being as my mother's Irish Catholicism came to the fore with litanies of my achievement.

Our tiring journey ended at a tidy, small farmhouse. A sweltering mid-June day in Jasper County, tender corn stalks opened, and early zesty tomatoes ripened in the perfect weather for growing a rich harvest of fruit and vegetables. It wasn't a day for city people like my mother, who despised humid heat and only found solace with her instant electric fan and cool breezes from nearby Lake Michigan. I caught the scent of newly mown hay and saw Uncle Fred. Sweat-slicked dark hair pushed under his old felt hat, he arrived with his heaped wagon of fresh feed for the two horses.

"Let's get started," he said. "We've got a new litter of pigs, mama cat had her kittens, and Betsy dropped her calf last week. Be careful of Butch here; that collie is one cranky dog with all that fur in this heat."

Ecstatic, I breathed in the farm and smelled the wonders of sweet grass, mud-caked pigs, overheated dog, dry cow manure, wilted garden flowers, and Grandpa's home-cured hams hanging in the smokehouse. The farm was Dad's pride and joy, I knew.

"Five proud generations of our family have farmed this homesteaded land," Daddy's sister, Aunt Ruby, asserted. "And each generation has made improvements in the management and yield per acre. Your Uncle Fred isn't kin, but he's the best farmer in the district. Everyone knows that."

I felt at home in Grandma and Grandpa's two-story farm home, which, strangely for our family, they shared with their daughter, Aunt Ruby, and her husband, my pal Uncle Fred. After all, in our suburban neighborhood, this blending of generations would never happen.

Aunt Ruby, pushing a bobby pin through her stray hairs, welcomed us with hugs and her usual chuckle. She enjoyed her brother Van's kids on our once or twice-annual visits.

"Poor Aunt Ruby," my mother intoned once, a distinct hint of her superior fertility slipping into her comment. "She had a bad case of uterine tuberculosis as a teenager and could never have children."

I grabbed Sharon's hand and obediently followed Uncle Fred, dragging my still-sniffling little sister behind me. Uncle Fred ignored the commotion and encouraged us to follow him promptly. Instead of relief, I sensed only outrage from my mother, who, still quivering from Sharon's near-death experience, had to tolerate the cautioning commands from Grandma, the visiting aunties, Madge and Cappa, along with Ruby, who joined in the warning chorus. Grandma and Grandpa said almost nothing throughout these noisy days of our visits, Grandma because she was overwhelmed and Grandpa because he was stone deaf.

"Don't even try to get near momma pig today," Uncle Fred advised. "She rolled over on two of her babies this morning, and she's in no mood for little kids right now."

Our mother decided to err on the side of vigilance, perhaps fearful that those country people would think she was a poor mother.

"Sharon, you get inside this house right now," Mommy commanded.

Dropping Sharon's hand, I rushed off, taking full advantage of my superior age to check out the marvels, leaving Sharon to sit on the kitchen baby stool, blubbering harder than ever. Too young to participate and excluded from petting the calves, holding a baby pig, or fondling the kittens, Sharon sulked in the hot kitchen, but to no avail. Somehow, Marilyn and I stayed under the radar of our protective family. Still, Sharon, cast into unknown dangers and never acclimated to farm life, experienced one catastrophe after another over our many visits.

One of our stays took a nasty turn for little Sharon. Pre-bedtime, nightly trips to the outhouse invariably had an ominous feel. Without the moon's glow, the darkness quickly overshadowed us. We staggered slowly along the path, lacking proper lighting to guide the wary traveler to the tilting outdoor privy, long overdue for a cleaning. On one occasion, we left the flashlight batteries on the kitchen sink back home, so we were out of luck for an electric aid. Mommy and Sharon would have to brave the trek alone.

While they fumbled through the weeds to the outhouse, I lost ten consecutive foot races. I never ever won, not once, to my over-energized father. I am a poor loser, running the other direction from my gloating father and throwing my twelve-year-old self down on the browning front lawn. Rolling on my back, I paused to watch the glorious flight of the fireflies. Suddenly, I heard shouts from the outhouse.

"Help, help, come right away!" Mommy shrieked into the gloomy night.

The next moment, I heard Uncle Fred's heavy steps first on the front stoop, then rushing past the well and around the chicken coop, he lunged toward the far-flung outhouse. Cries from Mommy and Sharon mixed with the clatter of boards as I stood to join my father.

"She'll be all right," soothed Uncle Fred as he carried Sharon inside. "Her little bottom will be sore for a few days."

"I just stepped outside for a moment," Mommy laments. "She fell in, and I couldn't get her out!" Mommy didn't tell them that she stepped out to light a cigarette.

"Well, she's out now, Alice," he replied as he set Sharon down. "Needs to be cleaned up, though."

Uncle Fred always seemed to know what to do.

From then on, my fed-up mother began her slow burn that ate away any interest in farm life. What filled me with joy loaded my mother with anxiety. For my lace-curtain Irish mother, the injuries of the place were legion: the smelly outdoor privy took the top complaint, followed by the horrendous smells of animals, the flapping, squawking chickens that hovered outside the front door, unfashionable furniture, and the lack of electricity. Next in line for annoying included an unpredictable corn-cob kitchen stove, a battery-run, static-ridden radio, and ever-blackened kerosene lamps. Everything seemed to throw her into fits. And only boring farm news the entire visit!

None of us loved the dirt roads that covered the house inside and out with dust, nor the massive horde of flies swarming in the kitchen and sometimes trapped on fly paper. Still, I knew we could endure all the hardships, the rural setting filling me with joy. As for the antique corn-cob oven, I discovered it produced an array of mouth-watering treats: award-winning cakes, pies, and succulent yeast rolls that melted on the tongue. Though rough, the oven was at least equal to the Magic Chef gas stove Mommy bragged about at home. I felt terrible our mother could not embrace this place I loved.

The rural neighborhood farmers, their older sons and wives, and the hired men gathered at one another's homes to harvest peak crops of oats or corn, an event Dad anticipated with relish. The occasions were not unlike family reunions or church suppers, as the farmers exchanged lively stories and gossip and looked forward to a bountiful noontime feast.

Summer signaled the first harvest time for swapping help as the grain crops matured—usually mid to late August. The second harvest came in September and October when corn was pulled off the stalks by hand and shelled from the cob. Never wasted, the cobs became valuable cooking fuel. Uncle Fred took the crop to a grain mill where they ground it, then traded the grain for livestock feed.

While the men worked in the fields, women cooked the entire morning, frying chicken, cooking potatoes, stewing vegetables, slicing tomatoes, and baking bread and pies to prepare for the 9-12 harvesters. Promptly at noon, they waited in line at the well. Taking turns at the pump, they vigorously washed their faces and hands with a bar of sudsy Ivory—soap supplied by Mommy, who could not tolerate the smell of Lifebuoy, the usual offering. They rinsed themselves with the chilly water and wiped the water off with flour-sack towels Ruby provided. After a long morning, the men were hungry and tired. Still, they had God-fearing souls and were never too weary of forgetting to say a communal grace and never at a loss for politeness.

"Thank you, Ruby. You and your sister Cappa are mighty good cooks. We sure appreciate you ladies serving this tasty food," they would say.

After the men had finished and moved outdoors to talk, smoke, and rest up for the afternoon of arduous labor, the women and children sat down to eat.

"Whoever invented all these meal items for a noon dinner that takes all morning to prepare and most of the afternoon to clean up?" Mommy muttered quietly under her breath, her frustration driving her into non-stop complaints.

After the outhouse incident, she began to fixate on keeping Sharon in one piece, leading to excessive restraints on my freedom.

"Don't let her out of your sight; keep her away from all the animals," she directed. "No more accidents." My unfortunate mother hunched on a wiggly kitchen chair, trying to get comfortable. Restless, she fanned the relentless perspiration that flooded her face. "Especially, don't let her touch that filthy collie," she whispered. "It's a disgrace."

I bit back my frustration as I realized that my full-time job now was to look after Sharon. Oh, why did I have to take care of that sniveling brat of a sister? Staying clear of the dog was the last straw.

I adored the dog, hugging him tightly at least five times a day, worshipped every other animal sight and sound, and found farm activity fascinating. There had to be a way to get around this debilitating duty. I dragged Sharon around in a squeaky old wagon when she was still small enough to fit. Later, as an emerging teenager, I took her in secret to the barn for meetings with my hero, Eddie, the newly hired man, a robust, deeply suntanned fellow in his late twenties.

"Tomboy!" the aunties called to me. "Take off those pants and get back into your skirt. Act like a lady."

I waved them away, skipping out from under their adult alarms, and trotted back to the barn or wherever I could find Eddie.

In my endless search for independence, I escaped from the adult kitchen crowd of food talk, gossip, and censure, when given half a chance. Eddie represented everything I craved: freedom, outdoor access, and physical strength. In my imagination, he was an icon of male adulthood I could neither resist nor overcome. Eddie was not a local boy but a drifter out of Kentucky without family or friends. His education stopped in third grade; farm labor was all he knew.

Over two summers, I became infatuated with the hired man, hanging out with him for long summer hours, sometimes helping, more often hindering, his farm duties, much to the dismay of my parents, uncle, and aunties.

"Nanette, you're taking up too much of Eddie's time," Uncle Fred said.

"You're gone all day. What are you doing with yourself?" Aunt Ruby chimed in.

"You're not spending enough time helping out. Your mother needs you," Aunt Cappa declared.

"You're getting rowdy and misbehaving. Stop it right now!" my father shouted.

In making my getaway that second summer of self-emancipation, I learned the art of bumptiousness—ignoring adults, sassing parents, running up and down stairs, and banging doors. The farmhouse vibrated with my excessive motion while my relatives' dismay and anger grew, especially after Uncle Fred found Sharon wandering in the milk shed unattended.

"You're shirking your duties, Nanette," said the worried adults as Fred carried her back to the house.

"If that cranky cow hadn't bellowed," he said. "I don't know what would have happened to Sharon. She'll have to stay inside now."

I felt no remorse. Instead, I wanted to experience more freedom than ever to move around the barns, hen house, and cornfields.

Our perilous adventures with Sharon continued, especially after I eluded adult control. In one too close to call episode, Uncle Fred and Dad took Marilyn, four-year-old Sharon, and me to the nearby swift-current river to swim. When I tentatively stuck a toe in the water, Daddy took the opportunity to promptly throw me in over my head into deeper water, his usual way to teach me to sink or swim. I bobbed to the surface, struggling to breathe, and paddled my way against the current to the bank.

"What's the matter with you, Nanette?" Daddy laughed. "Two summers of swimming lessons, and you're still like a fish out of water."

He reached for Marilyn, who immediately shrank from his touch. Uncle Fred lifted his hand.

"That's enough, Van," he said. "The current can take someone away quickly."

His words were barely out when I glimpsed Sharon. She had wandered off again to play on the muddy shore below. In a flash, she slipped, lost her footing, and fell backward into the fast-moving water.

The men seemed to act in slow motion, staring at one another as the deadly water rushed over the gasping child. The rapid current threatened to carry Sharon's small body to a stony end while Marilyn and I stared transfixed, trembling in terror.

Uncle Fred moved first. Kicking off his shoes and undoing his belt, he sprinted down the slippery bank and plunged into the mid-June, still-cold waters. Uncle Fred's strong swimming moved him beyond the current, enabling him to snatch her hair. He put his arm around the neck of what looked like a ragdoll and stopped her motion downstream. His quick action salvaged the shocked, still-sputtering child. Dragging her to shore took only moments, then he gently lifted her and made his way through the muddy bank to the safe grass above.

Daddy, overcome, threw up his arms, then whacked his hips.

"Oh, my God!" he yelled as he stormed off to the car.

Sharon would spend a lifetime avoiding water, except for her two suicide attempts as an adult, in both instances jumping from the Burnside Bridge in Portland, Oregon.

After the near-drowning incident, my father's patience fell to a low ebb. He became wary, vigilant, and irritable. His beloved rural life had become a menace to his suburban wife and children, casting a shadow on future visits. His critical eye fell exclusively on me for the rest of this visit. Perhaps the episode with Eddie that led to Sharon and the surly cow was too much for him to bear. He started to call me out for any minor mishap—being impolite to Mommy, not finishing my work detail, or even speaking out of turn. I felt his constraints tighten. No one was on my side anymore.

My resolve to escape heightened. I felt sure Uncle Fred warned Eddie to quit hanging out with me, and maybe Eddie warned me too, but I refused to budge. I remained willfully disobedient. Eddie became my only refuge, and I took full advantage of being with him every spare moment.

Then the dreadful day came: 6:00 a.m. I dashed to the barn expecting to see my heart throb finishing his milking, but instead, I confronted a stern Uncle Fred.

"Isn't this too early for you?" he said blandly. "Better get back to the house and finish your breakfast."

"Where's Eddie?" I demanded impatiently. "Isn't the hired man supposed to do the milking?"

"He doesn't work here anymore. I fired him yesterday."

Stunned, I can't believe this adult treachery. Where did he go? Where could I find him?

Beneath the adults' silence and glowering stares, I felt a hopeless sense of loss that nothing could undo. Not only had I lost my best buddy, but also, I had betrayed my father. For a moment, I bore his unremitting shame since I'd dishonored Daddy in front of his beloved relatives.

I slipped into his raging regard, freedom gone and covered with insults as my father began his invocations of "stupid" that went on for months, even years; I suspect his remaining lifetime.

"You're stupid," he'd say to me. "You did that stupidly. Why do you act so stupid? You must be stupid. There you go again, Miss Stupid."

"I hate stupid people," he muttered, the most punishing remark. Putting me in place became his overarching position. "You're too big for your britches. You'll have to settle down, and I mean down. And no backtalk, do you hear me?"

So, I returned home at thirteen years old to dull domesticity, plodding school life, and an overfull household of four children, including Davey, the prized boy, toddling around under Marilyn's tutelage. Sharon seemed to have been forgotten in a rush to welcome this long-awaited male addition.

I reined in my energies, taking the two flights of steps one at a time instead of skipping steps to the bedroom level or into the unfinished basement. I carefully hung my clothes and the other children's outdoor wear on designated hooks (which they promptly pulled down). I scrubbed floors and bathrooms for my mother's bridge days without protest and phased into becoming my mother's lady's maid. At the same time, my father's list of demands grew exponentially, all delivered in a thundering voice before his morning departure, with all tasks completed by 6:02 p.m., the time of his return from the city.

Poor Mom, how would she survive without a maid after sad, overweight Mae and the half dozen other country girls vanished when better opportunities came along? Reading became my only escape with long school and evening work duties, without friends, and even forbidden night-time radio listening.

Meanwhile, Sharon faded into the background, no longer accident-prone but suffering the consequences of safe behavior: no one paid attention to her. The cherished brother occupied the family's notice, casting Sharon further into the shadows.

After our grandparents died, the farm took on a different complexion. The long-awaited New Deal rural renewal program heralded a rapid evolution out of subsistence farming and animal husbandry. It transformed the land into mechanized agriculture, single crops, and commercial development.

When we returned to the family farm for Uncle Fred's funeral years later, I confronted a barren landscape with shock. Aunt Ruby sold the five-acre oak tree section for lumber. The buildings suffered massive bug infestation from bird loss due to pesticide poisoning. The topsy-turvy winds left the air hazy, spreading cloying dust on mouth and clothes. The soil smelled of pesticides, the chemicals had killed the butterflies, and the once-so-abundant chirping birds, now silenced, all disappeared.

How could the countryside's splendor have vanished so quickly?

CHAPTER FOUR

Loss

Sharon's tribulations "settled down," in Daddy's words, once we returned home from our most recent country ventures. We resumed our family's suburban lifeways and left Sharon to sink again into the quicksand of obscurity.

One early wintery afternoon with icy conditions that made for precarious walking, Daddy drove slowly up our narrow drive to the smallish but well-designed 1930s garage. He eased himself out of the car, walking on the ice-skating rink he'd built earlier that season, carrying a blanket-wrapped, squirming bundle. As I watched from the window, I wondered what was next.

I heard him nervously stamp his snowy feet on the porch mat outside the kitchen door. Then, striding into the kitchen with a hearty grin, he proudly presented a miracle—a beautiful, curly-haired, long-eared, black cocker spaniel.

"Here's a gift for you, girls," he said proudly, "born on the Jewish holiday of Yom Kippur (my father was a stickler for special days), so we'll name him Kippur. How's that?"

He turned to my mother, who stood scowling in the background. She seemed only concerned with what the newest charge would require of her attention.

"And he's not a mutt," Daddy replied to her unspoken question. "You'll be happy to know he has a full pedigree with papers."

Why he thought that information would assuage my mother's worries about doggie mess—urine, hair shedding, and noise—remained a mystery. Her frown continued as the children clustered around him and the precious miracle.

Daddy never flinched in the days and weeks that followed as I took over dog care. He barely finished patting Mommy's arm when I reached out and claimed Kippur for my own, despite my sisters' making cooing sounds behind me. I held onto the impression that my father meant to make the dog mine without the necessity to share him with my sisters. I suppose I should have been kind and shared Kippur with Sharon. I could feel her disappointment and exclusion, even as I clutched my cherished puppy.

My trouble in school and on the playground—excessive nervous behavior, inability to focus, and irritability—led to a parent-teacher conference. The nuns seemed alarmed at my lack of sociability and withdrawal and expressed concern about my grades dropping and disinterest in learning.

My father's musings may have been something like this. What does a parent do? A dog could be the answer. A dog could bring me out of myself; give me something to care for. After all, Dad always had dogs and one or more pooches trailing after him, whether working or hunting.

Whatever his reasoning, I embraced Kippur as my sole responsibility.

"Ohhhhhh, I can't believe it," I gasped once the puppy was in my arms, my heart sticking in my throat. "The best present of all."

We fell in love instantly, Kippur and I, in what I trusted would be a lifelong companionship, a happy blending of an eager, face-licking, tongue-lolling, wiggly puppy and my best self. After much coaching, Daddy and I set about to train and guide the new puppy into doggy adulthood. Neither Marilyn nor Sharon seemed interested in this phase of doggyhood, or perhaps I ignored them if they were, as I continued to treat the dog as mine alone.

Life is never that easy. First, the dog was not easily trainable by a ten-year-old. He made a ferocious mess on the carpets, not once or twice, but over and over. Soon after arrival, my sweet little dog took on a strange, beastly smell that my mother found offensive. She required me to bathe him frequently in the children's bathtub. Mom also demanded I clean up the hair and dirt he left behind, ensuring that the tub would have permanent rings my child's hands could not quite reach.

He lasted in my bedroom for less than six months before falling from grace. Banished to the basement, he languished in a room overloaded with broken furniture that my father said he planned to repair someday. Somewhere along with abandoned and unwashed clothing, the wringer washer, the mangle iron, and the clotheslines, Kippur found a place to rest.

When I turned eleven, I worked in the basement every Sunday afternoon and did the family laundry next to our loud, sinister furnace. The frightful clanging the furnace made when it came to life terrified the quarantined dog and initiated his howls of discontent. Rarely did a peaceful night go by without his nonstop howling. I prayed for his restoration to my bedroom, again sleeping at the bottom of my bed. Instead, matters worsened when my parents cast him out of the basement to an even more lamentable location: the utterly cold, unforgiving, damp garage.

My father assured me Kippur was in "doggy heaven" since he had a special door that swung open at a touch of his nose, a warm, cuddle bed with heaps of blankets, and a secure, late-model dog house, all inside a refurbished, cleansed garage.

"Remember," Daddy insisted, "I grew up with dogs, and none of them ever saw the inside of a house. Dogs have a way of adjusting to the outdoors. They grow a thicker coat of fur. Don't worry about him. He'll be just fine."

After hearing Kippur's heart-jerking moans a few nights, I accepted our common fate. I took my father at his word: the dog would survive, and I'd continue to miss his presence at night.

I gave myself over to loving Kippur. I lived to play with him after school, before bed, and early in the morning. We frolicked together in the winter snow, on the lush summer lawn, in early spring dawn, rain or shine, whatever the season, laughing, singing, and talking dog language. Kippur often uttered noises of ecstasy as I rubbed his tummy and exchanged his licks with my kisses. How could I have known this idyllic state would never last?

The day began like all others: rushing to dress, eat, feed Kippur, and romp around the yard. I dimly recall my mother calling me shortly after feeding the dog. Of course, I must lock him back into the garage, race the three blocks to church for daily Mass and communion, then march in single file into the classroom to quickly find my desk, and sit at attention until Sister calls for the first prayer. A typical start to my school day.

"Don't forget the note for your teacher," she said, causing me to spin back to the house to pick up the note, but left the fence lock undone. While in class, Kippur was on the loose, entirely on his own.

Hours later, Mommy told me she received a call from the veterinarian around noon.

"He told me a car hit Kippur in front of his office," she reported, still rattled. "The vet managed to fix him up. He'll live, but his badly mangled leg requires him to amputate. The doctor wanted to know if we wished to put Kipper down."

"I told him 'no, absolutely not. My husband will take care of it,'" Mommy insisted.

My mother immediately called Daddy, who abruptly departed from his office, enduring the tiring hour-long ride home from Chicago to the suburb, then a quick exchange of greetings, information, and money between the two men. Soon Kippur arrived at the house in a large box and again plopped into the dark basement to await my arrival from school.

Kippur eventually healed but was never completely restored. It took many weeks for him to learn how to walk again and then to adopt a lopsided run to keep up with my bicycle. I marveled at how seriously he took his lessons; my commands barked loudly to demand his full attention.

"Good dog," I said. "You're doing so much better. Even when I race the bike, you're keeping up. You're so special, Kippur, so special."

Sometimes he would forget his absent limb and trip, slowing our progress, as he accompanied me on various fast-paced jaunts around town. Those daily skirmishes with a girl, bike, and crippled pet went on throughout the summer into the fall, with rarely a day passing without a breathless outing. Despite his disability, malodorous scent, and too-frequent whimpering, I loved my sweet cocker spaniel. His eyes followed my every move, his expression undergoing every change of mine, and his doggy mood mirroring my own.

Cold descended from Lake Michigan in its most bone-chilling wind blasts that winter.

"At five below zero before Thanksgiving, it'll be a record this year," the radio announcer proclaimed. Despite such dreaded news, our basement, with its furnace warmth, could no longer contain Kippur, whose sounds of misery resonated through the house. My sleep-deprived, practical parents banished him to the garage.

Unfortunately, the move only made matters worse. The dog rendered howls of agony in higher octaves, long-drawn-out, wolf-like wails that penetrated the neighborhood. How long could this last, I reasoned, before Daddy brought the dog back and let him sleep with me? I was confident Kippur would quiet down once he returned to my bedroom.

Then again, I failed to consider adult reasoning: my mother's refusal to share her home with a despised pet and my father's conclusive way of settling matters. This rarely (or never) involved reversing a decision and never planning to inform the children beforehand. Nighttime calls from indignant and irate neighbors persisted for days until my father finally moved to take care of things decisively. His plan? Alleviate once and for all the gloom-and-doom situation caused by this three-legged and parent-rejected creature.

One blustery March day, the wind shimmered over the lake, reddening my exposed legs, tossing hair around my head, and leaving me breathless. I set out to my first urgent stop after school: to let Kippur out of the garage to play. I imagined him throwing his entire doggie self into the swirling air, but when I opened the door, the sounds were missing: no happy yips and scrabbling across the floor to meet me. No dog at all.

"Mom, where's Kippur?" I called. "What's going on?" I searched the garage, becoming more frantic with each moment.

No dog, blankets, leash, only minute traces of him were left, mostly his smell. My mother did not answer my questions.

"Did he get hit by another car?" I pressed. "Did he run away? Did Kippur die?

More silence, a silence so heavy I could drown in it. I ran to a few of the neighbors.

"Have you seen my dog, the black cocker spaniel with three legs?" There was even more silence, but I saw disgust sweep the neighbor's face.

I studied my father's withdrawn face as he entered the kitchen at his usual 6:02 arrival time. I could see he had news for me—bad news, horrible news, the worst news in the world for a 12-year-old.

"I had to put the dog down," he said plainly. "I didn't have any other choice."

Kippur suffered, both Dad and I could agree. Still, I could not accept him destroying my dog. Killing the smelly, stump-oozing animal that other family members mostly ignored became a dark deed to my childish thinking.

I felt a heavy melancholy settle over me that lasted for days, weeks, and months from that moment into late winter, spring, and then summer. With the grief came a mounting frustration and horror at how something I loved so dearly could be snatched away, to disappear—hardly to heaven. My dog's life ended without mercy by a swift, deadly injection. Was I the only one to grieve him?

If only my father had talked to me before doing the deed. If only he had explained the necessity of relieving the wretched dog's suffering. If only I could have prayed over my loss before it happened, and especially, if only I could have said a weepy goodbye to my beloved friend—then I could have been more at peace with myself—and stopped hating my father.

I believe that my father was not by nature a hard-hearted man. Practical, yes. Overwhelmed, on occasion, yes. Trying to do the right thing, yes. He could even be gentle and kindhearted. I sensed his deep pain when he delivered the sad news to me at age twelve. When his much-cherished mother died that same year, he felt stunned. We held each other, both weeping for our losses.

CHAPTER FIVE

A Father's Struggle

My father's life was shaped by hard work and worry over money. Born in 1901 and growing up on the Illinois prairie, his people farmed the acreage for five generations. There was no haven for farmers in this heartless world. Van revered the land but knew the tragedy of crop failures. At the tender age of nine, he fell off his favorite horse, Ben, and stretched out on the ground lay inert, immobilized with pain. Unable to move, it was hours before anyone looked for him, let alone rescue him. Heavy farm work further weakened his back, permanently damaged his sensitive colon, and delayed his education until adulthood. He remained shamed by his name (Dorris) and his ongoing physical weakness. Yet, ever adaptable as a teen, he took on his middle name, Van, and began strength-training exercises.

He completed the one-room schoolhouse lessons in a few years. Still, the shortage of farm hands—especially after his older brother, Verdan, abandoned the family and headed West for a "real job"—crippled further efforts to pursue formal training. At age 21, he decided to ride his dilapidated bicycle nine miles to attend Newton High School. He quickly moved into the ranks of scholar, debater, and class leader. Upon graduation, he embraced the urban world as his own.

About five hours by car from Jasper County, Chicago beckoned thousands of young farm men like my father, promising employment and opportunity. The business and management courses at Northwestern University drew him in further, and the scintillating atmosphere of Chicago opened up opportunities with its nearly anything-goes mindset.

Introduced to Alice by his new and dear friend, Clarence (her brother and chaperone), they soon formed a threesome. Captivated by her spirited disposition, engaging laugh, and accomplished Charleston dance steps, Alice came to represent the new world, far removed from the emotionally blunted, plain-Jane farm girls of home.

After a year, Van asked Clarence for Alice's hand in marriage, as was customary in Catholic families of that era. Clarence hesitated, knowing his deceased father would have been unhappy with his daughter marrying a Protestant, but Van's charming and intelligent manner won him over.

Hired full-time as a salesman and newly married, my father carefully stashed money in not one but two banks, believing this to be more prudent. With only an ambivalent attachment to the city, he planned to build a new home away from Chicago, reflecting his temperament as a man of the soil.

The second bank crash of 1931 occurred a few weeks before I was born, an unrelieved financial disaster that deeply affected my father and millions of other small savers. His dollar dreams evaporated after the first banking crash in 1929. He felt confident that his second account would carry him through to pay the obstetrician and provide extra help for Alice while she healed from my difficult birth and learned how to care for a baby.

After my birth, he became more cautious, placing his savings in Woolworths' company plan, which could never fail unless the company collapsed. They neglected to tell him that Woolworths had a poor reputation for returning savings if an employee left for another job.

Like many *Chicago Tribune* readers, Dad blamed Franklin Delano Roosevelt for the shabby way the government treated him and all the other ills of the Great Depression. I suspect he secretly believed he should have bought Illinois black-soil farmland instead of putting his hard-earned money into the "damn unpredictable Roosevelt-meddling bank system."

A job in the clothing industry turned out to be a lifesaver. Dad rose in the ranks of the company while his relatives sat in the gloomy darkness of their farmhouses, kerosene lamp fuel long used up with little cash to buy more.

Dad, always generous, shared what he had with his parents and sisters and provided financial assistance to Alice's widowed mother. My Grandma's sons ignored my father's request to assist their aging mother, yammering twiddle and twaddle but never giving a penny.

We girls adopted his desire for independence and witnessed our mother's judgment of men who lacked dad's drive. How did these family values affect Sharon, who longed for and never attained independence?

People admired my father. We all did. We were in awe of our Dad; I know I was. An impeccably dressed, well-spoken man, he was purposefully competent and an imminent problem solver. His capacity for charm could not be overstated, making him the most successful salesman in his company. He enjoyed taking care of business.

"Trust Van with financial matters," said his supervisors with approving nods.

His smooth exterior came at a price. Even in his thirties, Dad's worried expression marked his features with furrows. As he aged, the lines lengthened, giving his face a strong, squared-off, Pioneer-American look, much like his ancestors, whose old photos my sister Marilyn collected from various relatives, now long gone.

I wondered how a man moving from a confining homestead niche in mainly impoverished rural Illinois could make a life-changing shift into the hard-driving, big-city life and later into the affluent suburbs. He had to have been a very astute, discerning man to learn a different way of life. A life that included a four-bedroom home with frequent remodels, a live-in maid, four children in parochial schools, and a wife who failed to grasp the enormity of the mental and physical effort it took to create a substantial lifestyle in a society only then emerging from the ruins of the Great Depression.

Dad's ambition soared, totally fixated on creating a beautiful, well-ordered world for his wife and children. My mother only knew her husband to be an outstanding, if exceedingly thrifty, provider. Mother often compared herself with her sisters, Betty and Marcella, whose husbands, Mom said, experienced frequent bouts of drunkenness and unemployment. What I noticed was my mother's shame about their poverty.

Even during the war, regular trips to the farm on hunting ventures and domestic animal slaughters of pork, beef, and chicken afforded our family the luxury of meat when most Americans, limited to their meat coupons, had so little. We only ate meat on designated days, though, keeping faith with wartime restrictions of meatless dinners to help our soldiers at the front.

Dad disliked cheaters and even told some of his neighbors they were unpatriotic Americans if he discovered they had falsified their ration coupons for food items or gasoline. Other times, he shared his largesse through gifts from the garden and built much-needed bonds with Protestant neighbors, suspicious of his Roman Catholic wife.

My father wrestled with his German heritage, despised during the two world wars, by calling himself Dutch or French Huguenot, replete with an entire history of a self-created ancestry. Perhaps, he encountered prejudice in his line of work or a verbal confrontation by a stranger during those war years. At home, he proudly pointed to Trexler Town, Pennsylvania, settled by the Pennsylvania Dutch in the early 1800s, as proof of his American loyalty, even though the same people were immigrant Germans who also rewrote their ancestry.

CHAPTER SIX

The Irish Catholic Contingent

Baptized Alice Margaret, our mother, grew from a charming baby into a petite, pretty girl with two bright bows in her black, glistening hair. She became her Daddy's favorite, cuddling up on his lap every chance she had while ignoring her overworked, tired mother. She even refused to learn how to cook or sew like her two older sisters.

"Daddy doesn't tell me I have to, so I won't," she would say as she fluttered her outsized eyelashes.

John Monaghan, her father, and Anna, her mother, had three older children: two girls, Betty and Marcella, and a son, Patrick Clarence. After Alice's birth, they had two more sons: Paul and Eugene. With blond-haired Eugene's sudden death at age two, devout Anna began her prayers of intercession, asking God to give her another son, and promised in return that she would raise him to be a priest, whatever the sacrifice.

"I will give him no choice," she pledged. "He will only be a priest."

Blessed with the miraculous birth of Dickie at the advanced age of 52, Anna enjoyed her life for a few years while John's insurance company flourished. Their two older daughters attended the state teacher's college while Clarence prepared to set the world on fire, becoming a successful business executive. Paul followed in his father's footsteps with an insurance career. Flighty Alice planned to attend junior college but seemed more taken with dancing the Charleston, wearing short skirts, and listening to the latest dance tunes playing on the gramophone. Little Dickie clung to his mother, obedient to her every wish.

When John died of a heart attack at age 56, the household fell into chaos. Forced to take on well-to-do clients to support her family, Anna sewed far into the night, sometimes muttering unintelligible prayers while pounding the treadle machine, straining every ounce of her energy. Determined to allow dutiful daughters, Betty and Marcella, to pursue their education as her husband requested, Anna ran out of funds to support Alice's junior college efforts. Alice plunged into the job market with only limited skills and never achieved the educational level of her sisters, a deficit our mother felt all her life.

Even though Alice never mastered stenography, that artificial office language, nor won any prizes for typing, she sparked up an office with her bubbly personality and infectious smile. She excelled at working the front desk, holding her own in meetings, and greeting employees and visitors alike. Later she would describe office work as a good place for her.

When Van appeared on the scene, Alice dazzled the love-struck swain with her smile, dancing, and scintillating conversation. With her brother Clarence as the official chaperone, Alice declared Van the perfect match: tall, good-looking, ambitious, and, according to Clarence, a "pretty good catch." Unfortunately, Van wasn't a Catholic, a grave concern. To circumnavigate this inconvenience, Alice made Van commit to raising the children Catholic, a promise he followed faithfully.

Alice's life made a quick turnaround after marrying Van. No more midnight agonies of hearing Anna's nightly thrust on the treadle of her worn sewing machine. Alice shook off the maternal slurs about her running around town, wasting money on clothes and lipstick, and otherwise acting unladylike. Her mother's cruel disappointment about Alice marrying a non-Catholic troubled her. Her Irish family, on both her mother's and father's sides, had a lifelong legacy of despising Protestants, even the non-British ones. The Protestants, they believed, brought Ireland low, created periodic famines, and forced loved ones to separate and flee their motherland. Although never spoken out loud, the resentment held firm in the older generation. Alice loved her Irish heritage but cared little about the history of British victimization of the Irish.

As a bride, Alice faced new responsibilities, and cooking became her priority. She lacked the culinary skills of her sisters, Betty and Marcella, so Van laid out ingredients, provided the recipes, and guided her through the entire process of creating a meal. Under her husband's tutelage, Alice learned quickly and became a superb cook. She even made fruit pies that Van declared excellent.

Van endured an irritable stomach and bowel problems that required more than average attention: no lard, uncooked vegetables, or tough cuts of meat. Like Van's other character traits, his eating habits tended toward the picky and perfect. A fatty cut of beef could shatter his well-being for days, as Alice learned early in their marriage. She willingly adapted to his special needs and, after a year of firm coaching on household management by Van, felt ready to start a family. She also called on her two sisters, who Alice asserted were very smart, both college graduates, and helpful for assistance with healthy eating.

However you define normal, our early childhood hardly seemed out of the ordinary. Our Mother attended to our childhood illnesses with diligence and care: temperatures taken, medical advice followed scrupulously, prayers offered at bedtime to protect our frail bodies, and heaps of praise given to the child who swallowed medicine without complaint.

Holiday rituals consumed the household in preparations and celebrations. Christmas, always a lavish affair with gifts for all, produced an overabundance of festive dishes—some years, plum pudding with rich vanilla butter sauce served as the culinary centerpiece. The house shone with radiant Christmas décor: tree lights and ornaments for the living room and gifts piled high under the tree, a holly wreath spread wide on the front door, soft candlelight shimmered, and a gorgeous Christmas bouquet on the dining room table all completed the glorious occasion. That is, until the children tore into the carefully wrapped packages, littering the floor and chairs with colored paper and their newly acquired loot.

I coveted action and mobility. Bicycle, roller skates, ice skates, and sleds were my treasures, all to my father's displeasure and my mother's misgivings. Birthdays, likewise, provided happy breaks from the routines of school and family life. New toys, precious books, cake and ice cream, and a child's favorite food made the day joyous. On some occasions, of course, our parents gave the wrong child a special gift, as in the case when I surreptitiously passed on an elegant art set to my sister Marilyn, knowing I could never change my "C" grade in that subject, regardless of how hard I tried. She, in turn, found the roller skates too daring an enterprise and showed relief when she handed them over to me. I'm sure my father often wondered if girls should be so lively and on the go.

Following Lent, forty long days without sweets, and after the tribulations of Good Friday—enduring religious services lasting three hours—Holy Saturday reigned with bliss and blessedness. On Easter, the Church's highest feast day, my Mother stepped forward as composer and conductor of a lavish early spring affair, creating a festival to remember.

We eager children gathered in the kitchen, ready for the annual Easter egg coloring with its assortment of decals—ducks, chicks, bunnies, flowers, and butterflies. We placed each decal tenderly against the egg, gently moistening and holding them in place for a few seconds until the dye set. Sharon fumbled with the slippery egg and giggled as the colors dripped into formless shapes. I achieved only blurry designs, leaving the artistic part to Marilyn.

Easter Mass, with its triumphant music— "Christ the Lord Has Risen Today," the glorious Bach cantatas, and more traditional Church music—lifted our hearts and minds into a place of wonder and grandeur. As usual, our father remained home from Mass, bereft of such blessings. After church, secular renderings on the radio: "Here Comes Peter Cottontail" or "Easter Parade," filled the day with rapture.

Easter dinner, often with relatives, overflowed with a lamb roast, casserole potatoes, new crop asparagus, and homemade pies. Easter bunny baskets, piled high with chocolate bunnies and candies, sat at each child's plate, waiting to be devoured after the bountiful meal. We children sacrificed our health and well-being to consume every bite of sweets before bedtime. Our mother's leniency, only reserved for special days, we knew could not last.

Mother shopped daily at the local grocery store, departing from the house after breakfast clean-up, walking to the corner of tree-lined Greenwood Avenue, and continuing for three blocks to the modern Gothic St. Joseph's Catholic Church for Mass and Communion. After church, she pursued shopping at the only area grocery store across the street from the church and rarely missed a brief stop at the bakery with its breathtaking aroma of fresh bread and sweet rolls. Finally, she would step into the drugstore for cosmetics and book rentals. At 10 cents a copy, she could rent two or three books for the week, enjoy captivating novels or thrilling adventures, and stay within Van's strict budgetary restrictions.

When we moved to Wilmette in 1939, I remember the grocery store cans and boxed items stacked to the ceiling. Mother would hand the clerk her grocery list, and he would scour the shelves, up and down, with his moveable high ladder to retrieve cans of tomatoes, beans, peas, peaches, boxes of Kellogg's Corn Flakes on the lower shelves, and Post Shredded Wheat cereals on the upper shelves. Then, we would move to the display cases for dinner salad items. Finally, the eager clerk would step behind the meat counter to cut the exact portion of beef or other meat she had ordered.

Fish materialized on Fridays when Catholic customers crowded in for their weekly sacrificial meal. Lake Michigan fish were abundant: whitefish, trout, yellow perch, panfish, smallmouth bass, and bowfin, as well as some species of lake catfish. After one of the children choked on a large bone, probably from the perch, our mother chose a whitefish filet with few bones for Friday dinner.

Once I turned nine, Mom and I acquired a new piano and a teacher. Mr. Rummel became part of our family routine, a tall, balding character who weekly taught mother and daughters the art of the instrument but never caught on to my incapacity to read music. I painstakingly memorized each song, and after dozens of lessons, I thought our teacher might get wise, but he overlooked my nearsightedness and ignored the well-memorized pieces.

Compared to my halting progress, our mother's piano skills ascended as she moved from simple beginnings to complex pieces. "Clair de Lune" was her greatest triumph. Her ear, tuned to harmony, picked up a vast repertoire of traditional and modern songs. Frank Sinatra's "Night and Day" and Duke Ellington's "Sophisticated Lady" were her favorites.

Sharon appeared to have an exceptional talent for the piano, one I could only envy. She knew notes, practiced regularly, and came out of her shell for rare public performances at St. Joseph's grade school.

Our mother had her most rewarding moments sitting at the piano, gliding her hands over the keys. Yet, the piano disappeared once she left Wilmette in 1967 for southern California after Dad's retirement. Was it a cruel loss or a sign of her inability to claim space for herself in the marriage?

Mother loved compliments and sought her children's approval at every turn.

"How do you like my latest fashion, this exquisite silk blue dress, girls?" she asked one day as she twirled her full skirt. Then turning her back to us, she bent her left knee and, with a provocative look over her shoulder, adopted the leggy pinup pose of Betty Grable, available on calendars for the troops during World War II. We, youngsters, sighed appreciatively and hoped we could look like Mom when we grew up.

My mother claimed vernacular speech as her own. I overheard Mom and Dad talking one night. He labored to explain why they couldn't afford a new refrigerator while she countered his logic with charming platitudes.

"Van, that's just 'penny-wise and pound-foolish.' You know, next year, it will cost even more."

I didn't hear his responses, only hers.

"'Better safe than sorry,' when it comes to appliances, we can't afford to have a breakdown."

There were brief pauses in her speech.

"'What will the neighbors say when they see that an executive can't afford to buy his wife a new, larger refrigerator?" she pressed on. "This 10-year-old Frigidaire has seen better days."

I imagined Dad throwing up his hands in frustration, her illogic invariably winning the day because soon after, a new refrigerator arrived, complete with all the best features.

Despite the loveable normality of these remembered scenes, a few oddities prevailed that affected all of us in my elementary years, primarily involving our Roman Catholicism. Our mother's religiosity and liturgical calendar dominated the household and largely determined our daily schedule from morning Mass to evening prayers—without my non-church-going father's comment. Our family stood out as one of the few practicing Catholic households in a neighborhood of Protestants. I recall the local boys shouting epithets like "papist" (for belief in the pope), "mackerel snapper" (referring to our fish-on-Fridays meal), and "mick" (for all those of Irish descent).

"Hold your head up," Mother would say. "Be proud of your religion."

Good advice, if you could dodge the occasional sticks and stones that went along with the verbal taunts. I have no idea how Sharon managed these confrontations with her gentle manner. Quite possibly, I took the brunt of these skirmishes since I spent more time outdoors than my sisters and had a more combative style. I suspect the effect on both girls was a take-no-chances approach of avoidance and withdrawal.

I noticed all my friends' mothers had sewing machines, allowing their students' compulsory school outfits to grow with the child. Matters worsened with Mom's absolute refusal to sew even a stitch, sometimes leaving us with tattered clothing: buttonless cardigans, hem-dragging school uniforms, and ill-fitting blouses. My uniform fit—for a while. It hung too long some years as I waited to grow into it; then, the outfit became too small in subsequent years. In fourth grade, I learned the art of the safety pin to patch up holes and rips and to put stray hems in line. My sisters were less fortunate. They looked bedraggled in clothes, often dirty and betraying a hint of neglect.

Mom couldn't be bothered to mend those torn clothes.

About that time, Dad realized the family required a seamstress, with order restored when he hired one. I no longer suffered embarrassment from classmates snickering at my sloppy array of visible pinnings.

I learned young that if I needed or wanted anything, the point person was my father. Reaching out to my father was a tough call since he was equally likely to say "no" as "yes," often at the whim of the moment. He invariably seemed to prefer the austere disciplinarian role when interacting with me. I knew Mom could be downcast by the overcritical and sometimes disparaging remarks he directed at her appearance, decisions, or conduct. She always tried so hard to please him.

CHAPTER SEVEN

A Mother's Decline

When did our family's life leave the ordinary and careen into crisis mode? Even before I became my mother's steady confidant, I began looking after Mom when I was twelve. I can't recall exactly how old I was when my mother's drinking flipped out of control and went from social to addictive. I don't know what circumstances or situations undermined my mother's reason and common sense, leaving her helpless and the younger children bereft. I know I stepped forward and tried to fill the social and emotional gap, but my crude efforts were inadequate to stem the rising tide of chaos.

Questions abound. Could my father's absences while on the road as a traveling salesman or his gradual detachment in favor of demanding executive positions have signaled the grim beginning of her decline?

Another possibility: my mother's inability to drive confined her activities to church, grocery, drugstore, and bakery. Did her lack of range feel limiting, or was it safe for her, until she found another way to escape her confines? Eventually, she discovered that taxis could get her to the new Orchard Village Mall, and home delivery services could supply her wide-ranging needs, especially for alcohol replenishments.

I often wonder if Mom's loss of a full-time maid after the war could have been a leading contender for her decline. Dad often confessed to me about Mom's horror of housework and claimed that was the real story behind the drinking. Or perhaps, her lack of intimate women friends in a non-Catholic community contributed to her sense of isolation? Did she suffer from the suburban segregation that beset many women of that time, creating a ghetto of wives and children? Or could her husband's promotions, which spurred her to cultivate a wealthy and well-educated women's bridge set replete with elegant lunches and cocktails, have been her downfall? With the small reserve of junior college stenography training, was she ever really comfortable sitting at the bridge table with two PhDs and a lawyer? How successfully did she match wits with these brilliant women?

Trying too hard to please, she kept up the façade that she was like everyone else—that's likely a part of the story. The other ladies enjoyed their sips and left our home tipsy but quite capable of driving home; while my mother ended up blacking out, our family routines shut down for the remainder of the day.

I suspect Mother believed her heroine days were over after a much-delayed hysterectomy after the birth of a son. At 11, I accompanied her on the monthly, then weekly, visits to her obstetrician in nearby Evanston. The doctor said that Mom had a "high-risk" pregnancy and would need to be very careful.

"The odds for both mother and child are not that good," he admitted.

"I'm not sure what's happening with the baby," Mom confided to me as the train rocked gently over the suburban tracks. "The doctor doesn't understand why I want to go through with my pregnancy despite the fibroids. I told him God has planned for me to have this boy, just as my mother prayed to have a son who became a priest. I also talked to my confessor about this. He says I'm doing the right thing."

Mom firmly believed she was fulfilling her destiny. Even though she knew that with her medical condition—the fibroids continued to grow as the pregnancy proceeded—she could die with a full-term delivery. Despite the risk, I noticed how Mom's pregnancy brought a glow to her face and light into her heart. I felt her happiness and certainty that things would work according to God's plan.

My parents were jubilant with Davey's birth on July 23, 1942. Mother and baby both flourished without distress, reducing their worst anxieties.

My mother survived the ordeal, but shortly after delivery, she prepared for the removal of the tumors. With her uterus gone and ovaries removed, radical surgery had more than medical implications. Hormonal irregularities, loss of her reproductive capacity, and post-partum depression conspired to unravel her high spirits and dispelled her self-image as a still-beautiful woman in "the prime of life."

"I feel low a lot," she said to me. "Too much to do. I'm so tired. Davey is such a happy baby, and I'm grateful for that. But I can't keep up with your Dad. I have these terrible hot flashes and night sweats. Look at me. I'm gaining weight. Your Dad can't stand pudgy women. Some days, I can't manage at all. Do we have some gin around? It's so hot outside. I think a gin and soda with a twist of lime sounds great. Better yet, please make me a dry martini. We've got some vermouth in the storage area." At age twelve, I did my best to follow directions, knowing this was not the right thing to do.

Once my mother discovered the quick pick-up of alcohol, she became a devotee. Unlike her beloved, alcohol-free father, my mother did not take the Catholic pledge of abstinence. She did not acknowledge the destruction of generations of Irish ancestors' souls who were obliterated by chronic drunkenness and unreconciled early death.

Usually compliant with her husband, Mom snapped back at the mere mention of her unruly behavior. Not once did she perceive her "social-only" drinking as problematic or question her singular opinion of being in charge of her life, the kind of avowals even her children knew were wrong. Our masterful father could say little to curtail the downward slide.

"I'm on the right track," she retorted. "I can keep my martinis down to two. You're wrong. Drinking's not my problem. Maybe it's yours. You mind your own business."

But, of course, two martinis earn four, four earn six, and too late, we would find her slumped under a table, draped over a couch, or just fallen somewhere. Mom's defeat signaled her husband's marital but mainly squelched outrage, his anger projected on someone else or something else: the government, high taxes, Democrats, a child.

As family conflict heightened, Sharon hid in her bedroom, holding tightly to herself as she rocked back and forth in agony.

In a moment of reckoning—and Mother surely must have had a number of these—she would decide to go "on the wagon," but a week or two of sobriety was all she could manage. I often wondered why she didn't seek the consolation of our nearby church with its austere but trustworthy priest, Monsignor Neuman, and the five junior acolytes who served the congregation. Once I came of age, and for my mother, that was age 16, she talked candidly about her feelings of alienation from the local parish.

"I have nothing in common with these German priests," she lamented. "The parish never feels like home to me after my Irish parishes, like St. Tim's or St. Henry's, with their friendly, cheerful priests. They're cold, these Germans, not sympathetic; they don't really care about me. I wish I could attend St. Francis across town. The pastor is a riot, second-generation Irish, full of love and laughter. But the diocese stands firm against switching churches. Oh, why did I have to end up with these Germans?"

How could she overlook her husband's German descent or neglect his need for order? Why was she blind to his rational thinking over emotional expression or his relentless quest for success goals, which he pursued with such intensity? He sought to exert his Germanic spirit of strength and stoicism, loyalty and protection, verging into sternness, to rule over his wife and household. Her father, unlike her husband, had an easy Irish charm.

Alice turned away from her husband's differences—class divide, ethnic-religious divide, gender divide, temperament divide—and the unresolved issues. After all, Van asserted his Dutch heritage—Pennsylvania Deutsch/German—mind you, not German at all. A weak claim, to be sure, yet it covered up a despised nationality during the war years. Dad also laid claim to the Irish side, his mother, and her kin, although his father's German influence held sway. My mother perceived none of her beloved father's softness in her husband.

I knew Mom needed help. I could hear her crying in the bedroom during afternoon "naps" and even in the bathroom. I needed to stand by her side, assist her in our tiny kitchen as she prepared meals, be ready to clean the dining room and sinks after we finished dinner, fetch her cosmetic bag or nail polish, keep the bathrooms sparkling. and harass the younger children to help out. I felt obliged to do these tasks because our father's unfailing requirement for order necessitated that I step up to the job. None of the children, especially me, seemed aware that such a state of affairs did not constitute an ordinary suburban family.

Undoubtedly, the neighbors viewed me as a model child as they observed my steadfast and daughterly devotion. Mom and I shared the fun of her music, and we gabbed together like buddies. We made a pact to keep Daddy happy without sassing, but I knew I fell short of this impossible promise. The neighbors did not see that the household hummed with dissatisfaction and lost opportunities, and Mom's unhappiness spilled over to me.

"You're late! Did the nuns keep you after again?" she growled one afternoon. "Your Dad's shirts need ironing. He went to work the other day with a dirty shirt. And you can't save ironing until the weekend. Too bad about your plans for Saturday. I don't like those sassy girls you run around with anyway. They look like troublemakers."

I bit back an answer. The week before, I overheard Mom humming an old Mother Goose rhyme, the one where an overwhelmed mother commits child abuse.

There was an old woman who lived in a shoe.

She had so many children she didn't know what to do.

She gave them some broth without any bread.

And whipped them all soundly and put them to bed.

Instead of lashing out in anger as I might have expected, she sighed.

"That's how I feel, Nanette," she admitted, "like the 'old woman in the shoe,' so I'm glad you can look after things while I rest. God gave me a good girl. I feel so worn out sometimes."

On other days, Mom loved making promises.

"Let's have a picnic tomorrow," she said. "We can go to the Village Green. They've got plenty of picnic tables. I've picked a great spot near the spreading maple tree."

I learned not to trust these promises.

"OK, next week, we'll all go to the zoo," she would say. "It'll be fun. The *Tribune* reports the zoo has a new baby elephant."

Nothing came of these avowals for special outings.

"As soon as your Dad comes home, we'll arrange to go to the Forest Preserves for a day. You and your Dad enjoy playing ball. You both have beautiful skin and get great suntans. I must stay out of the sun or get those ugly red blisters. But there's plenty of shade for the other kids and me."

Along with broken promises came the extended afternoon naps.

"I'm tired," she whispered once through a slit in the bathroom door. "Keep everyone quiet. I'm going to bed now." Her afternoon application of cold cream oozed gently down her clammy face.

How could anyone sleep so much on a meltingly hot August day with not a breath of breeze?

"Mom, it's already two o'clock, and you said you'd take us in the taxi for ice cream."

"Don't be a nuisance," she replied. "Your Dad's left change on his bureau top. Get some ice cream when the Good Humor Man comes along. There he is now. Hear the bell? It makes my head ache, ding, dong; it's too loud. Tell Marilyn Davey can't eat chocolate."

We children held our breath those summer days until she emerged from her bedroom. But at five sharp, she was up, freshly bathed, wearing a frilly cotton dress, and often "ornery," as Aunt Ruby would say.

"You haven't picked the peas yet," she'd tell me. "I know it's hot, but your Dad wants creamed peas tonight. You know I can't be out in the sun with my skin condition. I'm tired of talking to you. Just do what I say. And pick up that messy game the kids left all over the living room floor. You know he'll have a fit if he sees that."

More than a nag for clean-up, our mother could be completely unwound by our dad's displeasure at the disorder.

Marilyn seemed to be the frail one in the family. I remember she often had to stay home from school, which irritated Mom if Marilyn had additional needs. I recall an episode that, in retrospect, seems too dreadful to dredge up. Mother, now taking tranquilizers after her hysterectomy and ovariectomy, had been behaving erratically that morning. She shouted at Marilyn from outside her bedroom at some point. Nine- or 10-year-old Marilyn either failed to respond, or our mother couldn't hear her.

From my bedroom down the short hall, I heard Sharon scream from the other bed, and what I saw was unthinkable: our mother holding Marilyn in a sitting position, was stifling the breath out of the sick child. Enraged, Mom had rushed into the bedroom, where Marilyn was crouching under the covers, and grabbing the pillow under her head, stuffed it into her face, muttering something unintelligible.

I must have pushed Mom away, grabbed the pillow, and said something I thought my father would have said in his tone of voice. "That will be enough of this." I know I walked her out of Marilyn's bedroom and back into hers, urging her to lie down and rest until she felt better. What could I have said to Marilyn? Probably nothing. We had been taught to overlook such happenings.

CHAPTER EIGHT

War Years and Beyond

This chapter is an imaginary letter to my sister, Sharon, describing shared family dramas over six years. These memories recreated 70 years later reflect the stresses, strains, and high points of our growing-up years.

*　　*　　*

Dear Sharon,

I felt sorry you were treated like the lost lamb in first grade that Monsignor Neuman always talked about in our St. Joseph's grammar school catechism class. I knew our father was too busy, and our mother, too tired from her pregnancy, was cranky. We sisters seemed to ignore you, and even the dog, Kippur, sometimes pretended you weren't there. Of course, Mom loves you and, once in a while, would pat the top of your head, saying in a soft voice,

"Poor little Sharon."

You know, we all loved you. You were such a cute little kid with those big blue eyes. But not much more out of Mom. What I'm saying may sound harsh, but maybe Mom didn't pay much attention to you because she thought you were too little to help and in everyone's way.

That year, 1942, was tough on the family when the draft board notified Dad of his draft status: 1A. What disastrous news for a 41-year-old family man! He could have been called up for enlistment anytime. They were looking for men with a college education to serve as officers, and he fit the bill. The war went on longer than anyone expected, with a greater chance our father would never return.

I suppose you or Marilyn asked: "What will we do without our father?"

Our mother acted utterly distraught. "It's a disgrace to take a man with so many children. How will we live?" You both cried a lot; maybe, I did too.

Poor, nervous Daddy. He nearly hit you when your boots slipped out of your hands and left snow all over the hallway. I'm surprised because he never used to hit you or Marilyn. I asked for it, I guess. I sassed him back so many times. You were the good kid; you'd never have done that. Marilyn just cried, and that made Dad feel sorry for her. Even when he was at his most ornery, he gave her hugs. It looked like it made him feel better.

Mom was plenty worried during those final months of her pregnancy. With Daddy waiting for the draft and Mom having all these medical problems, no one was very happy in those days. A few months later, it was a different story when Mom finally had the baby.

"A beautiful bouncing boy," she said.

"What a relief," we all said. We knew Mom had a lot of pain and was terribly sick.

Still, she was overjoyed and kept repeating, "We finally got our boy. God answered our prayers."

Dad had only one thing to say: "No more babies for this house."

You may have been too young to remember, but little Davey was more than the cherished, long-awaited son. His birth freed our Dad from the threat of military service since men with four or more children received exemptions.

Sharon, I knew how unhappy you were to hear that Mommy needed a critical operation after Davey was born to ensure no more babies. We prayed together, and see, our Mom turned out OK.

* * *

When you entered the second grade, Mom sternly said, "You're not a baby anymore. You need to pick up your clothes and hang them up."

That happened after we lost our Russian maid, Olga, who barely spoke English. Mommy hired her about nine months before but couldn't stand her mouthing off. You used to run upstairs when Olga went on one of her tirades.

"The only thing I *have to do* is die!" Olga repeated for anyone to hear.

But the Russian maid captivated me, and I started spouting the same thing. The day Mom asked me to help in the kitchen, I played it for all it was worth. With hands on hips, I snapped, "The only thing I have to do is die—and I won't do those dishes or anything else I don't want to." I thought I was so clever.

Well, you saw what happened then. Daddy grabbed a stick, so I ran outside into the front yard. I thought I'd be safe, but he followed me out there, grabbed me hard, and hit me with the stick all over.

"When she sasses her mother, she'll get the stick every time," Daddy said.

Thanks for feeling sorry for me, though. I've got huge cuts all over my legs and back, and I couldn't stop screaming. I could hardly stand up when he finished. I hated it because all the neighbors could see Daddy hitting me right there—in front of everyone. I don't remember who was out there, but people could see what was happening. You were wise to get out of his way.

Remember, it took me three or four days to return to school. I appreciated you staying home with me on one of those days. Sorry I didn't enjoy the board games you tried to have us play.

The day after Dad beat me up, I overheard him saying to Mom: "Maybe now that Olga's left, Nanette will settle down." That comment just made me mad.

Thanks for coming to my aid and telling Dad that I was too old to be pushed around. I felt grown-up at 12 years old, always at Mom's beck and call: helping her out with the housework, running to the store, or anything else she asked me to do. Olga wasn't any good, anyway. She was always complaining.

Mom told us our Dad's angry because he works himself to exhaustion, never letting up. "Do you notice how he brings his briefcase home every night and works at the dining room table for hours without looking up? He worries about the job, but he frets mostly about money. I think it makes him sick," our mother said. She worried about his health.

"Your father has a bad stomach problem and needs to rest much more. That's why he stays in bed on the weekends so often. His stomach is upset, and his back hurts too, so he can hardly move."

Then I told you he had colitis and some kind of irritable bowel problem with diarrhea. I think you asked: "how do you know this?"

"I'm snoopy, that's why. I liked going through Daddy's papers in his brief-case, the ones in the closet, and on his dresser. Once I found a sexy novel, along with his medical papers, in that closed case—the one on the top closet shelf in the hall. It's remarkable, but I never did get spotted. I went through that bag so fast; I read everything. I expected that any time I'd get caught. And you must have said, "I'm sure glad it's not me."

When Dad was really sick, Mom insisted. "Don't irritate your father." Keep quiet, don't talk, and stay in your rooms when he's sick."

I thought then: Wouldn't you think he'd like to have his kids visit him when he's in bed? Sometimes, I did it anyway. I suppose I bothered him with my questions and occasionally sassy remarks. And did you ever say when I kept pushing on Dad? "What's the matter with you? Can't you just shut up for a change? You'll get us all in trouble."

You acted scared that Daddy might hit you, so you stayed out of reach.

Mom didn't seem to mind too much my bothering my father. She liked spending time with me talking about "girl stuff." Maybe she pretended we were sisters. You must have asked me why our mother didn't speak to you like that. I found an excuse for her: I'd tell you it's because you're still too little. Certain things upset Mom, especially when Dad was too busy to talk to her, housework, bills piling up, and many other things. Then, she went after Marilyn, said mean things, and sometimes hit her. Why does everyone around here hit little kids? Of course, nobody smacks Davey. He's the golden boy; everyone loves him. He has the biggest birthday parties anyone had ever seen, especially the one when he turned five that hot July in 1946.

I still reminisce how much you loved Halloween and "trick or treat." I thought it was babyish, but Mom regaled us with her story about how Irish immigrants brought it to America, complete with pumpkin carving and trick-or-treating. She loved to tell us that it was a religious holy day, "All Hallows Eve," which occurred the night before All Saints Day, a holy day of obligation on November 1. That's when ghosts, goblins, and graveyards open up with the half dead. I'm sure she scared you half to death. It's good our mother thought the holiday needed celebration so that you could have a little fun for a change and tons of candy.

When you were seven, I recall you wearing your bunny outfit and carrying your little basket around the neighborhood. I must have walked around with you, but I refused to wear a costume. I already had the dreaded sensation I was making a spectacle of myself walking with you in those weird bunny ears Mom couldn't quite get right. You were happy, though, "grinning ear to ear," our Mom said, as neighbors dropped candy and apples into your basket. In those days, she spent most of her time with her beloved boy.

When Dave started kindergarten, didn't he look cute in his new black pants, white shirt, and red vest sweater, the school uniform for boys at our parochial school?

"My little man," Mommy always said.

Everyone thought he was super handsome and loved him so much. It's too bad Mommy never said anything nice about your looks. And you said, "Maybe I'm *homely.*" *Homely*: that was our mother's favorite word for girls who aren't pretty. We both knew it was not a good thing to be homely.

I remember you used to play with Davey after school, but after Dad decided to have him do only boy things—Cub Scouts, Little League, or practicing ball with

Daddy—that left you out. Who could you play with? Marilyn had her art projects. I practiced every minute for the Marywood Academy for Girls school play or had my head in a book. I despised that school, Marywood, but Dad said to Mom:

"It's good for her. The nuns keep her in line."

I thought the nuns were mean, and I always told Dad that. At some point, he said that you never had to go there. You noticed Marilyn wasn't planning on Marywood when she entered high school. Dad permitted her to attend the public high school like the non-Catholic kids in the neighborhood. And you followed Marilyn the following year. You wanted so much to be popular; everyone wanted to be popular in high school.

I fooled everyone. Even though I went to an all-girls school, I had a line-up of boyfriends and managed to go out every Friday and Saturday night. Mom thought it was funny that I had lots of dates with different boys, especially that former neighbor kid I used to play soldiers with when I was 10 or 11. He was tall but kind of a creep. And I recall whining about his monstrous pimples. I only wanted to date the flashy kids and maybe college guys.

I had a hunch you never wanted to be like me, as Dad grumped, "giddy and stupid about boys."

Our Mom thought it was funny when the dates came over and waited for me while I fixed my hair and *slowly* put on make-up. She'd play the piano super loud when the boys stood at the front door or jiggled on the chair, waiting. Sometimes the dates had been drinking, but Mom ignored it and sipped her cocktail while she ran her skilled fingers over the piano keys.

We sisters all had the impression that Mom believed we needed to be pretty and admired and we'd get by. Dad always pushed for good grades.

You told me you thought you weren't as smart as Marilyn and me. Worse, you thought you weren't as pretty. And you moaned to me a couple of times about never being popular. I couldn't believe it when you said, "Maybe I'm a loser, like the 13-year-old girl in my class who stupidly got pregnant and had to go away somewhere."

Why would you ever think that? I suspect Mom said something to make you so anxious. She constantly compared us to movie stars, neighborhood girls, or each other. She used to brag about me looking like Elizabeth Taylor. What a crock! I think Mom was full of exaggerations, don't you? I know I laughed it off, but I sensed it made you feel not so pretty.

It made me mad when Mom used to say you weren't popular because you were a "shrinking violet," "little mouse," and "a wallflower," which had to make you feel like one of Dad's limp, dying roses.

Dad made me work, first at the factory when I was 14, boxing up the caps and gowns eight hours a day, and the following year at the office. It wasn't fun and games for me, popular or not. Dad's idea was to keep me in line. He used to say:

"She has to dress up and stay quiet and take orders. Nanette needs to learn a thing or two about the real world."

He never said that about you or Marilyn. Maybe he thought you two didn't have to learn much about the real world. I loved the attention at work but was always tired and cross with Dad's driving from Chicago to home.

The trip back home from Chicago to Wilmette with Dad was no picnic. He liked to blow his top after all day at the office. Oh boy, what a difference. I saw him calm, smiling all day, and even flirting with his lady employees. The minute he got in the car, it was a nerve-racking experience. But I'm stuck with it. I had to work until school started again in the fall. Some of it was fun, though. I got complimented for my fast typing and being an errand girl, bringing coffee and donuts to the workers. Everyone smiled at me and said, "what a wonderful girl."

Did you shudder when I said this? It seems it didn't sound like much fun.

* * *

Do you remember the day you were 11 years old, and Mom finally bought you that journal she promised you? You had one page for every day of the year. Oh, how you loved writing in it. Dad even suggested you use his office paper and write anything else you wanted for each day. You told me you started with a story about your piano lesson. The music teacher, Mr. Rummel, thought you had a natural talent and urged you to practice more. But as I recall, Mom liked to get on the piano stool the minute you came home from school, and your practice time was cut short. I'll bet you wished you could have sassed back like me and gotten her off that piano stool.

Do you remember having that terrible day at school the winter when Dad was gone a lot and Mom and I were at each other's throats, keeping everyone awake? Dad told us to be careful about telling anyone. We had to keep it a secret because Sister Henrietta, your sixth-grade teacher, nice as she was, asked way too many questions.

"Don't tell them anything they don't need to know, especially the nuns. Next thing you know, it's all over the school."

He meant the bad stuff at home.

We both realized Mom was never at her best when she started drinking when our Dad was out of town. It was always my job to keep things together, so I stopped it before it was out of control. The worst day was when Mom had the four big bottles delivered from the liquor store, sometime after dinner, around 7:00 p.m. I lit into those bottles, opening up one after the other and pouring them down the kitchen sink. One after another, after another, after another. That was enough liquor for all his annual sales meeting dinner parties! What a waste! Daddy would have had a fit. He must have known about it but never said a word, at least not to the kids.

Mom screamed and yelled. She even pounded on me, but I didn't flinch. I suppose I looked funny. I still feel my cheeks all red and puffed out while I cursed a blue streak. Naturally, you were scared, so you dashed upstairs to hide. Marilyn had your bedroom door locked, and wouldn't let you in, so did Dave, and we could never go into the parents' bedroom—ever, ever. I declared my room "sacrosanct," and you were too frightened to defy me.

I caught a glimpse of you sitting at the top of the steps and waiting until it was over. You couldn't stop crying. I knew things were out of hand. What could I do? Dad expected me to take care of business when he went out of town. Did I make matters worse? I suppose you and Marilyn wondered why I had to be the big boss just because I was 17.

But nothing deterred me. I was determined to make Mom stop.

"Mother," I screamed. "I'm reporting you to Dad. This is disgraceful, and I won't have it for a minute. He told me to keep things under control here."

But Mom wasn't taking "no" for an answer. She shrieked back.

"Nanette, stop, stop. I promise I'll go to my room and be quiet. Just don't throw any more liquor into the sink."

"OK, Mom, one last chance. You haven't eaten any dinner, and you'll be very sick if you start in again with the drinking. I'm doing my homework on the dining room table to keep an eye on you."

How can you forget? Mom rushed up the stairs, pushed you back on the top step, and yelled.

"Get out of the way, Sharon!"

Then you told me you hit your head, and Mom headed for the bedroom, slammed the door, and dialed the liquor store on the new rotary phone. Naturally, she orders another batch of whatever it is she drinks. The delivery guy, Herbie, the liquor store owner's son, who knew Mom, showed up 15 minutes later, and it all started up again. Mom and I continued to battle it out, even worse this time. I'll never forget my anguished outburst.

"I will smash every bottle that comes into this house! You can bet your life on it!"

But too late. Mom met the delivery guy on the driveway, and he opened up a bottle right there for Mom, and she started gulping it down. It was damn good it was nighttime, so the neighbors didn't see it. None of us could believe how drunk she gets! After the rest of the bottles were inside, I was crazed in the worse way, pouring the remains of one bottle and the contents of the two others into the sink, smashing bottles, screaming, crying, and cursing. Poor Herbie ducked out fast before I started my most enormous commotion. I felt terror over what Dad would say or do. I never planned to tell him a thing about this outrageous situation.

You know the story. Mom won the battle, after all. It took me half the night to clean the mess up, do dishes, finish my two essays for school the next day, and try to get some sleep. I also cut my finger pretty badly, picking up all the broken glass. After Mom went to bed after the last fight, I breathed. Finally, the whole house sighed, peaceful and quiet after that terrible hullabaloo.

You poor thing, Sharon, you said your head ached all the next day. Too bad you couldn't use your journal writing for a school assignment. Oh well, we both knew nobody would believe you, anyway.

What a family we are!

Bundles of love,
Nanette

CHAPTER NINE

Victory and Defeat

The Victory Garden was a community-organized, privately financed acreage that was popular during WWII, offering residents the opportunity to grow fresh produce in a time of scarcity. Cherished by my farmer-at-heart father and envisioned as our would-be family collective enterprise, the garden effort lost ground quickly. Mom balked at physical work, insisting it ruined her nail polish. My artistic sister, Marilyn, had little hankering for the stoop labor involved, while Sharon was determined to be too young to handle tools. I became Dad's official garden partner, cultivating and tending the precious plants that fed our family through the war years under my father's stern direction.

The same situation held for food preservation.

"Too hot, messy, and exhausting," asserted my mother, who despised the tasks of peeling tomatoes, skinning peaches, or shelling peas. Pregnant with my younger brother, Davey, she could not stand for any time because of the excruciating pain of the fibroid tumors growing ever more prominent along with the baby. Dad never pressed her about helping out.

"Canning," mother declared, "should be kept for farm women or maids, not for my delicate hands and body."

After my sisters blinked and ran out of the kitchen, my father enlisted me to help him. Mae, the long-suffering maid, hampered by age and obesity, helped only with sit-down preparations. When it came to canning large quantities of food, she announced she had a sick stomach topped with a migraine headache. Dad shooed her out of our tiny kitchen space.

"More bother than she's worth," he muttered.

In the dog days of August 1942 and 1943, Dad and I sweltered over scalding water that boiled over the top of the kettle to sear young hands, stinging through the thick layer of zinc oxide. But can the homegrown produce we did. We filled dozens and dozens of Mason jars with fruit and vegetables, mostly from our Victory Garden and the farm in downstate Illinois.

We lined up the jars in even rows on dark storage room shelves Dad built to house the vittles: peaches, pears, beans, tomatoes, cabbage, beets, and peas. My father, ever the competitor, compared his grand collection with the sparse achievements of his neighbors and even his three sisters, the hard-working Cappa, Madge, and Ruby, whom he loved and admired so much.

Dad eventually recognized a better alternative after I seriously burned my right hand. Following weeks of study, he shifted to the freezing method after two years of canning. We were the only household on the street with an oversized freezer bursting with game pheasant, down-home beef, plump chicken, succulent pork, and fresh garden produce.

Despite my garden compliance, Dad and his farm relatives still considered me "rambunctious," a word I later found dates back to the 1830s. It refers to children who can be challenging to manage, overly energetic, wildly boisterous, and noisy. I fit the bill precisely.

Or at least they were always telling me that. Where I failed was my inability to fit into my father's expectations, requiring that I have a more stable character or at least one that obeyed in an always obliging manner. He thought I should have yielded easily to his will on every occasion, even *before* he expressed his intentions. My submissions proved a temporary oasis in a series of swirling sandstorms. He remained alert for signs of defiance, ending his sense of order.

Our father pressed ever harder to achieve the position of sales manager, and vice president, under the most trying circumstances of wartime and postwar product shortages. The limited availability of salespeople to take the products on the road and a president whose birthright was company ownership and advancing alcoholism caused Dad to become caustic and punitive. He irritated easily, snapping at us children, and invariably targeted me if I was anywhere in his presence. My father's struggle became our family struggle and may have laid the groundwork for future crises among family members: Mother's alcoholism, Sharon's mental illness, Marilyn's sudden-onset illness, and my adolescent acting-out behavior.

As the office situation accelerated, my mother found it increasingly difficult to tolerate my father's intensity, competitiveness, and work ethic.

"He never relaxes," she said to me, starting a familiar litany. "He drives himself continuously, and I'm afraid he'll get ill. And then he has that stupid golf league all day Saturday. Sometimes, he isn't home all weekend."

She openly feared for his health, but I imagine her inner truth told her that he was withdrawing from her. Perhaps she felt lonely, even abandoned. She frequently was troubled with hives, outbreaks that covered her body in angry red welts. Is this the period when she began severe drinking to blot out the growing distance from her husband? Or maybe her alcoholism emerged a few years after the seeds were sown in those absentee years.

Our parents, long convinced of Marilyn's fragile constitution, woke up to an unexpected health crisis. On a cold November day, I heard Mother's piercing scream that shook me out of one of my rare reveries to run to her rescue.

"Do something," she screamed at me. "Marilyn is shaking and shivering. Look at her face. Oh! Dear God in Heaven! She's fainted or dying. I can't stand it. Take care of her!" Mom bolted down the stairs and out the front door.

I did the ordinary thing in our household when faced with disaster; I called my knowledgeable father at the office. I calmly described what was happening.

"She has a bad case of the winter flu," he said, his voice clipped. "Listen to me very carefully. Put cold washcloths on her forehead and the top of her head. Wrap her warmly with blankets, give her a large glass of water, and help her get into bed. Above all, do not startle her! She's running a high fever. Call the doctor. The number is in my top drawer in the small black phone book."

"Thanks, Dad," I said before hanging up the phone. For a moment, we were a working team dedicated to a single cause: the family's well-being as Marilyn endured the first family flu of the season. But the teamwork did not last.

My adolescence and my non-stop resistance proved to be his ongoing curse. At the age of fourteen, I took another step into bold self-assertion. I threw away the object of six years of dental torture: the old-fashioned, steel-wire braces binding both upper and lower teeth.

"Where are your braces?" he demanded once he realized what I'd done. "You have another year to finish before they can come off."

"I don't have them anymore," I said, my jaw jutting defiantly. "I told you the wires hurt my mouth. I can't talk or eat with them. I hate them! I asked Dr. Lieberman to do something about all the bleeding, and he just shook his head. I've had those on for four years. I've had enough! So, I threw the braces in the garbage can last week."

"You did what!"

I refused to back down from Daddy.

"I found out Dr. Lieberman isn't an orthodontist," I persisted, "and he has no other patients with braces. He was doing it all as a favor to you."

"Don't be ridiculous," he roared. "He's the finest dentist in Chicago. Where did you hear that nonsense?"

My mother shuddered, quietly agreeing with my comments. Over the past few years, Mom and I discovered that Dr. Lieberman was a no-nonsense, no-Novocain, lots-of-pain-to-strengthen-your-character guy. I always felt beaten up after sitting in his uncomfortable dental chair as he drilled or banged away at my mouth.

"I asked him, Daddy."

"You asked him what?"

I stared at him in silence.

My father didn't appreciate the truth about his favorite dentist.

"Dr. Lieberman doesn't have the credentials for pediatric dentistry," I replied.

He closed the conversation, unwilling to continue the charade, and I was forever free of the affliction of wearing braces.

At fifteen, adolescence ruptured the last remnants of father-daughter peaceful coexistence. In his eyes, I appeared over-active, disobedient, and absorbed in other matters. I possessed an abbreviated attention span that effectively tuned him out. Once partners, our relationship dwindled into screaming matches, the dining room a battlefield of two combatants and timid bystanders. Repeatedly sent away from the dining room table with an unfinished meal, any "sassing" on my part churned out mountains of additional chores. My mother wrung her hands but had no voice in the matter.

"You're as stubborn as your father," Mom faulted me. "Keep quiet, and he'll settle down after a while."

I was especially tired of his half-hearted invitations to race on the lawn, play ping pong in the basement, or fool around with Chinese Checkers and other board games on the dining room table. Ruthless, he refused to allow me to win even once. Was I ever the victor in these unfair matches?

I suppose I made the same demands on his pocketbook as my school friends: expensive tuition, spending money, new clothes, and athletic outings that took me away from my family. He found it all irritating, as it stirred up anxiety about rising costs. More than ever, he needed my assistance to keep his wife under guard. The house felt rife with discord, jangling the nerves and generating undercurrents of anger. Her bridge party drinking sorties left her incapacitated for cooking and household management, the situation worsening without a full-time maid.

The once reliable help had fled from our household into higher-paying factories and offices.

He continuously charged me with *his* impossible goals, neglecting to ask me *if* I could accomplish them.

"What! You bring home a 98 percent grade in these easy courses of history, English, and Latin," he yelled one night. "That's not good enough in our family; you should have 100 percent on all your work as I did."

Assigned to weekly grass cutting, I dutifully ran the heavy lawn mower up and down the 150-foot backyard, pleased with my straight lines and the intoxicating smells of newly cut grass. However, my father's inspection of the results left no doubt I missed the mark again.

"You can never do it right, can you?" he railed. "This lawn is a mess. What are those crooked lines and missed patches of grass doing by the porch? It's an eyesore. This job must be done with precision. You will run that mower back and forth again and again until not a blade of grass sticks up. After that, rake all the loose grass and distribute it around the roses. And don't injure any of the rosebuds. Hurry up, your mother needs you in the kitchen."

What was the use of trying? Nothing I did pleased him. I refused to behave like a lady. I had run-ins with the nuns at Marywood High School for Girls. School became daily torture with new mandates to limit the students' span of personal control.

"No make-up, ladies," came a stern voice one day. "You heard me."

"But Sister Frances, that's not lipstick," I pleaded. "It's tinted Chapstick."

"You heard me, Miss. You'll stay after school again today and write a three-hundred-word essay on the principles of obedience that you can't seem to follow."

Dad had demanded I fertilize and water the rose bed before dinner, and I'd be two hours late to get home. I winced. You couldn't win at my school. I wanted to go to New Trier, the public high school, where everyone else in the neighborhood went.

I already knew the answer to why the nuns picked on me. They had determined that any child from a "mixed marriage"—Protestant and Catholic—could not be trusted. My father insisted I needed the extra discipline the Catholic school offered. They would not stop looking for excuses to put me in my place. I felt doomed to live forever in frustration. A bubble of anger threatened to choke me. I would find a way out, but the interminable high school years seemed endlessly filled with agitation from home and school.

My father often put me in fight mode.

"You will eat every bite off that plate," he said, "or you'll be sent away from the table."

"I cannot and will not eat those burned vegetables," I replied. "And those squishy oysters in milk broth make me puke. No, I won't eat that."

"I didn't ask what *you* wanted," he replied, his voice cold. "You eat what's on the table, Miss. Who do you think you are while I'm working like the devil to support you? Leave the dining room table this second."

I endured yet another long night of hunger pangs.

My father made use of various techniques to invalidate me. His favorite was calling me "stupid," to which he added sharp or angry responses, glaring or severely disapproving expressions, and abrupt dismissals achieved with a wave of the hand. Throughout my childhood, I had more than my share of slaps, hits, and spankings, harsh discipline, all of which were quite normal for a period when societal expectations demanded children be under tight control.

My teenage self strenuously resisted all these forms of discipline. I grew weary of ducking his swats across the top of my head and shoulders, of feeling like running away, and of looking for an escape where I could hide and be alone with my books. I felt worn down by an overwhelming sense of dislocation and loss. Eventually, my father's every command and even recommendation became suspect. I rejected them all.

Ours was a divided family. By the time I was in high school, our family of six had dispersed into alliances, relationships that excluded Sharon. The following diagram conveys how these relationships worked. A solid line indicates strong bonds between members, whereas a broken line shows loose bonds. For instance, our father and Marilyn had a close relationship, while Marilyn and our mother had only loose bonds. The difference is significant. My mother's over-identification with me, her eldest daughter, often had unhealthy consequences: my mother behaved as a teenager, flirting with my dates, over-confiding in me about her relationship with my father, and when drunk, acting infantile.

Nanette—Mother

Nanette- - -Father

Father—Marilyn

Marilyn- - -Mother

Marilyn—Davey

Davey—Father

Davey---Mother

Nanette—Marilyn

Mother- - -Father

Nanette- - -Davey

To offset my father's antagonism, I developed a secret passion: reading movie magazines with fan letters for our favorite stars. The Frank Sinatra craze captured my attention. Adopting the "bobby sox" look with rolled-down socks, tight jeans, and hyped-up behavior, I became "president" of the Frankie Fan Club. My favorite stunt was sneaking away to downtown Chicago—a route I knew well after going to the dentist—to see Frankie's live shows.

I must have generated some outlandish lies to spend nearly an entire day away from home. Maybe the family found my absence a beneficial lull and decided not to quiz me too closely. Dad didn't buy my tall tales and pointed to the mountain of incomplete jobs he saved for me. His disapproving look no longer had the slightest impact on my new, cherished persona as a rebel.

These and other self-willed behaviors contributed heavily to the standoff between my increasingly demanding father and my growing belligerent self. Certainly, I was too often the brunt of my father's harshness, which could hardly pass muster as part of his otherwise brilliant and strategic self. Why did he so quickly lose control and take the low road of anger, verbal abuse, and overly vigorous physical whippings to keep me in line? I wonder how Sharon felt watching Daddy push, shove, and slap me on the slightest whim.

I suspect my father perceived me as the typical "disobedient daughter"—a dreaded prospect for a female. Perhaps he thought: How can a non-compliant woman survive? Who would marry such an outcast? She could quickly become my financial liability, a lifetime drain on my patience and pocketbook. My daughter needs to learn her lesson before it's too late. There is no place in the world for a defiant female. Conform or die, alone and unloved. Perhaps he thought he was doing me a favor, clipping my wings to keep me submissively earthbound.

As for a solution to punitive parental authority, I continued to act out the teenage rebellion role as the first generation of post-World War II "smart-aleck" adolescents. Dating older boys, slipping out at night, and running with the public-school gang exposed me to a different world: parentless houses with large stashes of alcohol, beach parties with casks of beer, and combative sex with various boys in their father's overpriced cars. I tried it all with little satisfaction.

Ultimately, I did not tolerate the alcohol and found beer had a disgusting taste. The boys had become quite tiresome with their pushing and prodding. None of them could maintain a conversation for more than a few minutes, mainly because their drinking led to a nearly unconscious condition. By the summer of my seventeenth year, I was at my wit's end to find any significant purpose in being a rebel but lacked a more people-pleasing role.

Where was Sharon in all this family strife and change? How did she respond as a witness to the drama of our father and me acting out our tumultuous relationship?

Without a strong bond with any family member, I remember Sharon remaining mute and unseen, a victim of the unresolved conflicts of generations past playing out in present time.

CHAPTER TEN

Chore Girl

My own life felt pretty rocky, as well. Friends couldn't visit me because chores piled up. Play days ceased to exist for me in my middle teens. All my days were work days. Sunday afternoons, after Mass, noon dinner, and clean-up, I began the week's washing, hanging clothes, and ironing the linens with an old-fashioned mangle iron, caressing them into perfect folds to fit neatly into the closet. If the laundry were perfect, Dad wouldn't yell at me. If I spent too much time on it, I couldn't meet Mom's other demands.

Reviewing that period, I felt like Cinderella, cast away from the family circle. What were they thinking, sending a child of 11 into a dank basement for an entire Sunday afternoon week after week to do the whole family laundry? Doing those chores of washing in the old wringer machine, hanging all the clothes on the too-tall-to-reach indoor clothesline, and then mangling the sheets and towels was torturous. I couldn't even come upstairs between tasks. And the basement was damp, cold, and unfriendly. I remember gasping for breath. I wonder if that was the start of my asthma that has plagued me from age 12 through the present time. Only later in my teens did I get injections to treat the asthma.

I know I felt intense shame when I incurred frequent injuries. My small hands wrestling with the wringer produced sizeable bruises. Burns on my hands and arms from stretching sheets and pillowcases over the wide, mangle ironing board resulted in prominent red marks. I learned to cover up and never to reach out to anyone to prevent them from seeing my chore girl scars and ridiculing my appearance.

With his rural background, I can only surmise that my father was treating me as he and his siblings had been treated: life is work; there is no cessation; life will always be difficult; prepare yourselves. In Dad's era, children worked on farms and factories, made deliveries with horse and buggy, and labored at various dangerous jobs. That's the rural context he grew up in and observed throughout the 1920s and 1930s in Chicago, especially among working-class families. With her genteel Irish background, my mother lacked this experience but had a solid resistance to housekeeping. She was selfish that way. If my mother had protested my treatment, she might have had to do the work. And God forbid that should happen!

Children do not know the difference between maltreatment versus culturally acceptable behavior. In our suburban community, putting a child to work in adult tasks was not the norm. I knew that other children my age were allowed to spend their free time reading or playing games or spending time with friends. This allowed them to be more creative and easier going. The absence of friends and entertaining activities generated my discontent and later rejection of my father's constant demands.

Mom seemed oblivious to my bouts of sadness, irritability, and depression, but once I reported in as sick, she was back to being good ol' mom.

"What, another asthma attack?" she complained. "That's the third time this week. I'll tell your Dad to cut down that enormous cottonwood tree on the edge of the drive. It's affecting me too. My bridge partner, Andrea, told me the cottonwoods are the worst in years. I've called the doctor, and we have a 4:30 appointment for your allergy shot. You'll be fine in no time."

Our routine continued throughout my early high school years. I felt neither parent could get Marilyn and Sharon to do their share of the housework. I turned out to be an easy target for whatever needed doing. Some days I felt like I was turning inside out, spinning from a loving, amiable child into an angry, rebellious teenager. Encouraged by Dad, at 13, I took on paid babysitting jobs, freeing me for a few hours from the detested housework, and giving me a sense of independence. I started to assert myself with Mom when she became belligerent or overwhelming, but I did it to keep our buddy relationship going.

"Mom, I've worked all afternoon after school," I insisted. "I can't clean the kitchen floor tonight. Dad wants me to get a perfect score on the math exam. He's been tutoring me in algebra all week for this test. Couldn't I do it tomorrow?"

She slammed the refrigerator door shut, barely missing my hand.

"I know I'm not doing the floor," she replied. "That's your job, missy."

My mother's constant battle with housework pointed to an abrupt shift in standards of home maintenance post-World War II. The home as a refuge, transformed into the house of display, was pushed by gaudy television advertisements, where new household appliances, wall-to-wall carpets, and luxury drapes and furniture became the new middle-class norm. My mother's heavy smoking with overflowing ashtrays and collections of magazines, grocery lists, and various shades of nail polish on living room tables violated the new canon of an immaculate household. Along with my father's perfectionism, the dual pressures weighed on her. She could never seem to reconcile the contradiction of living comfortably and keeping everything tidy.

A few weeks after the showdown about the kitchen floor, I confronted her about the drinking.

"You started that booze before supper, and now look at you," I said. "Awful. Really, very bad. Dad's out of town, so it looks like I'm "it" to take care of things here. Now, look at you. You can barely walk. I am so ashamed for you, the shame you have brought on yourself. Please go to your room. I'll fix the kids' dinner and clean up."

Mom would have none of it, so we battled half the night. Determined to get her drinks, Mom pushed against my efforts to create normality.

I was too much on edge with my father, fearing his outbursts about Mom's drinking. My heart wanted to be an advocate for Mom, but my father's rage wiped out my compassion. I felt so overwhelmed when caught between them. I didn't notice how involved she was with my adolescent ups and downs, how she wept after Larry dumped me, how she rejoiced in my good grades, and how furious she was over the nun who knocked my grade down five points for missing one homework assignment. I started to blame Mom for everything. I guess we all did.

My religious life suffered as I missed daily, then Sunday Masses. I scoffed at prayers, too irritated to pray. School and home life pinched every effort to expand. My mother's drunkenness and disarray increasingly maddened me. My skin felt prickly when I saw her aggressive behavior toward Marilyn and her neglect of Sharon. Our buddy relationship soured, and I lied to both parents about my after-school activities. Even though I bonded with Marilyn, who seemed to admire my pluck, I ignored my younger sister and brother. I felt worlds away from their childish concerns.

For her part, Marilyn took Davey under her wing, and Dad spent plenty of time with his beloved boy once home from work. Sharon never seemed to get any special treatment, but what could I do about it? The weight of guilt grew as I distanced myself from my mother, slipping out of the good daughter role into some creature I grew to despise. I didn't want to disappoint either parent, but their clashing expectations made home life unbearable.

When I entered college, an amazing awakening occurred. Forced to live at home while attending nearby Northwestern University, I saw a clear contrast between what I began to recognize as an impaired family and the larger world of learning and skill building. As a middling student among a sea of dazzling minds, Marywood School for Girls had not prepared me for college academics. I needed all the time I could muster to keep up with my classes, an impossible task with the load of home duties. I dreaded returning home each night after days of feeling free and unencumbered.

At 20, after a nearly four-month shutdown following a sexual assault by a part-time boyfriend, I flew away to attend the University of Minnesota. There, I found myself and cherished my good fortune. I could even take a deep breath.

Soon after, I met and married Ph.D. candidate Jim Davis, whom I deeply loved and admired for his academic knowledge, kindness, and openness in accepting my splintered family. After a successful break from my family's dysfunction, I had a chance to create not only a new perspective but an entirely different, purposeful life. Still, I felt deeply sorrowful about my sinking mother, for whom I could do so little.

My conflicted relationship with my childhood home continued after marriage. On visits home with the children, I experienced unbearable stress that corroded my insides like battery acid every time my father deserted us, departing for who-knows-where and leaving me with my enraged mother. These trips exposed me to the old patterns, and I felt alone and without a friend. Jim rarely accompanied me because of his work.

The lacquered veneer of our lives often blinds us to the dry rot within. Over the years, I asked myself: could I have been there for Sharon? Could I have saved her from the muddle, the shouting, door slamming, pushing, shoving, slapping, and slippery slope we called home?

No, I could not have saved Sharon, protected her from the muddle, the stops and starts of our family journey, and the twisted course of her life. Saving myself seemed the only choice I could make then.

CHAPTER ELEVEN

Shotgun Daddy

D uring my high school years, my father had an annoying practice of greeting dates, who brought me in late with a fully loaded shotgun. How very humiliating! How utterly embarrassing! It was strictly an old country habit, which placed our family among the outliers. But one night, I felt nothing but gratitude for this practice.

When I was sixteen, Art, a sophisticated almost-neighbor, who lived two blocks away in the upscale Kenilworth neighborhood, invited me on a date, I quivered with delight. I chose my clothes carefully, just the right blue plaid, pleated skirt, and white cashmere sweater. The doorbell rang, and with my heart fluttering, I opened the front door, waved goodbye to Mom, and off we went.

I wish I could recall what event we attended, but I thought I saw my date pull out his flask a few times. It must be another sign of his high style.

"Why are we taking this back road, Art?"

"You'll see. There's a great view of the night sky you'll love."

I didn't love, once we parked, Arthur diving to my side of the car and maul-ing me, pulling my clothes off. I tried fending him off, but he seemed determined. After what seemed like forever wrestling with this drunk guy, I jumped out of the car and yelled at him.

"I have to tell you that my father will kill you dead if you so much as touch me."

Art laughed it off, but I repeated it. "Ask any of my dates. They'll tell you, my father is serious. The shotgun waits at the front door, and if we're late—and we are now one hour past my curfew—he is ready with the gun cocked. I'm warning you."

I began my long walk home, at least five miles. Art's car pulled up next to me, "get in. I'll take you home right now. But don't say a word to your old man." I was terrified. My clothes were in disarray, my hair mussed up, and one cheek burning where Arthur hit me. But sure enough, there was my trusted father at the front door with the notorious shotgun. When Art walked me up to the door, Dad looked at him and said quietly, "never, ever show your face around here again. Do you hear me?"

Dad told me the next day that Art, an adopted son, age 24, had long had a bad reputation, "a ne'er-do-well," he said. He had been upstairs when Art arrived and didn't get a good look at him, but once Mom told him who the date was, Dad exploded. Planting himself on a dining room chair by the front door, with his shotgun an arm's reach away, he waited for my return. I could never figure out how my Dad knew so much about other people and so little about me.

CHAPTER TWELVE

The Lotus Garden

The Lotus flower is an ancient and profound symbol of the planet and the human condition. Although rooted in mud, its flowers grow above the muddy waters, producing an exquisite blossom. In Christian mythology, it symbolizes the hope and strength of people struggling in their daily lives.

In literary practice, the lotus garden describes the context before things happen, all the details that lead up to the story. This chapter is my story of floundering in the mud and transforming from the experience.

I despised my life. Consigned at age 17 to a Catholic girl's school, dour-faced nuns governed our daily lives. Nipping at my heels like barking dogs, they kept me running in the direction of their choosing. I felt my existence shrinking to the size of a nut, a small girl squashed into the smallest possible space, leaving little room for breath or light.

A variety of teachers complained. "Nanette, sit up straight." "Why can't you follow the rules?" The homeroom teacher reported you late for gym class again." "What can we do with you? We're trying to save your soul while you bring trash reading material like that! Dear God in Heaven." "Your demerits have led you to our only recourse: bring your father in here once again to talk with Mother Superior."

And then I met Steve, my heartthrob. Brilliant, moody, super smart, a bit arrogant, sure, but a prodigy, handsome, a university guy majoring in science. Steve planned to follow his father into a physics Ph.D. and professorship. Well, Steve invited little me to attend the fraternity spring house party. Could I believe my incredible luck? Even more astonishing, my parents urged me to take Steve up on his offer with his older sister, Joan, accompanying me on the train from Chicago to upstate New York.

I was no match for Joan when it came to traveling. Joan brought her book, pillow, blanket, lunch, and treats. I brought dress-up clothes and high-heeled shoes. Nothing else. Determined to make a fantastic impression with my Sunday church-going clothes bought with money saved from my babysitting jobs, I lacked even a remote resemblance of a coed's wardrobe: pleated skirt, sweater, saddle shoes, and sloppy socks.

Once on the train, Joan ate her meal, chatting gaily, but failed to offer me a bite. She must have presumed I would eat my "picnic" later. Then out came the pillow from the efficiency bag, which she nestled snugly against the window, and proceeded to spread the warm blanket over her chilly body. Could I believe Joan slept the entire night until the train slid neatly into the upstate New York station? Hunger pangs and fear kept me from closing even one eye. What was I doing in this situation, anyway? I lacked even the slightest notion of how to behave—or what to do.

Once we arrived, Joan rushed out, jumping into her boyfriend's arms, and disappeared for the weekend. My date, heartthrob Steve, didn't quite make it to the station, sending a couple of his less-than-sober frat brothers over to pick me up in a rattletrap jalopy that looked ready to collapse. These unreachables embodied everything I ever wanted to be: brilliant thinker, talker, classical music lover, and advocate of high culture. What shall I do, say, act, and feel to get along with this fast crowd?

So, what did I know? I only knew I was desperately short of sleep, hungry, and fast approaching a state of terror. Where was Steve? Mr. Heartthrob was among the missing, still having not shown up by noon the next day to give me a welcoming embrace. Instead, he released me into the wilds of his fraternity mob in a sink-or-swim situation. I could run to the bathroom, bawling my heart out, or mentally square my shoulders and confront my fate: face up to this roomful of geniuses.

"You look lost, little girl," a frat brother said as he handed me a concoction that looked suspiciously like a martini (my mother's favorite libation). I smiled winsomely as he introduced himself as Jeff, who offered to squire me around while Steve finished his lab assignment.

Famished and thirsty from hours of deprivation, I swilled the offering under Jeff's approving look.

"These fraternity parties like to test who can handle their booze the best without flopping on their face. You're off to a good start, Nanette."

Only later I found the bar bill for that overly lubricated weekend cost more than $1,000.

Another drink appeared, and another. I became the center of attention as my now loquacious self bubbled out whatever inanities came out of my mouth. I thought I detected snickers from some of the boys, maybe eye-rolling, loud laughter from a few.

Jeff interceded with another martini, the bitter, acid gin, fresh out of the fridge, now smelling increasingly like puke and burning my tongue. Now, I laughed back, loud, very loud, as Steve entered the room and prodded me to tell my story, still without a hug. What story? I had no narrative to entertain these rude fellows who had put me in a no-win situation.

Gradually, their voices faded; the room became still. I had fallen out of the chair. Steve had lost his bet about my booze capacity to the sound of clapping, whistling, and foot stamping. The boys parted as an older coed rushed over to help me up, a staggering, exhausted child dragged into a darkened room, helped to bed, and covered gently by a quilt. I could feel the door closing and her whispering. "She's off limits," I think she said, leaving me to "sleep it off."

The "frat train," I was later told, operated clandestinely to take advantage of the less experienced, usually younger dates, leaving them physically and emotionally flattened by repeated sexual violations from these less-than-stalwart lads. And that's where I remained that dismal weekend without food, water, or solace, left behind, a sorry victim of a sporting game only these superior fraternity brothers could play. And they did leave me alone, unlike the other "green" girls who were not so lucky.

Once awake and very ill, I recounted my losses. Certainly, Steve, my 17-year-old crush, was gone forever. The frat brothers had made a mockery of my naivety, while the older coeds merely felt sorry for me—and kept their distance. I had allowed my self-esteem to be destroyed. Shame enveloped me. Could I ever lift my head again? I resigned myself to a life of misery. But before I could start wallowing in self-pity, my optimistic nature rose to the top. Sunk over the bathroom sink that Sunday morning, I clutched a cold washcloth on my forehead with trembling hands. Still groggy, I made four quick vows.

1. Never drink martinis.

2. Never drink anything alcoholic on an empty stomach.

3. Never attend fraternity parties anywhere or at any time.

4. Be a better example to my younger sisters.

It took a week to recover physically from that wounded weekend. It took months to rebuild a battered self and find a way out of the pit I had dug for myself. My father must have detected something was wrong, seeing my moping self draped over chairs and sofa.

"What's going on? You wanted to attend that college invitation but turned into Miss Sad-Sack."

I could see that his probing could release a dreadful outpouring, so I shrugged.

"No more frat parties for me, Dad."

Instead, I poured out my woes to Mom, our family counselor, who, even drunk, had an open heart for childish grief. She asked for no details, just letting me weep and agonize over my embarrassment, especially the loss of Steve. I had never known what love was before this moment until it evaporated like a summer cloud.

I learned something else in the spring of my great humiliation: failure follows failure in a stew of disasters.

I felt dismal after Marywood dropped me from the lead role in the senior play production.

I became disenchanted with school and learning and refused to attend my high school graduation.

I abandoned school friends and began hanging out with suspicious characters.

I rejected possible summer jobs and spent my days hanging out on Lake Michigan shores playing volleyball or finding pals with sailing boats, turning my skin into a horrendous shade of peeling sunburn.

I disregarded my parents and, in turn, took on my father's wrath. He continued his emotional abuse of non-stop name-calling: "stupid" and other put-downs—"stupid is as stupid does," "you're a real loser, you know," "you'd better shape up fast because I'm tired of supporting you." He convinced me that I had a botched life without a possible remedy.

My life, unmoored by family or trusted friends, teetered for two years in overload as I went through the motions of dating an endless succession of "cute fellows," as Mom called them, but unable to give my heart to any.

What I didn't know and couldn't know is that in this period of late adolescent ennui and hopelessness, I began to open my mind, heart, and spirit to suffering, a state of being never discussed, never even allowed to think about in my home. Empathy sprouted and grew and made real love and benevolence possible. But a few years later, it took an even more egregious situation to teach me these crucial lessons.

CHAPTER THIRTEEN

Reversals

Almost everyone has another side, my father no exception. His life, periodically sculpted by tender tokens of kindness and love, made allies of us all. Who could predict which side would face forward, though: the unkind, uncaring side or the kind, sometimes cheerful and affectionate one? I learned to be wary, biding my time until I sensed his underlying disposition. My mother knew his dual nature only too well.

Roses, for instance. Dad was obsessed with the care and nurturing of these delicate plants, undermined by biting insects, leaf-deteriorating black mold, and heavy rainstorms. In the summertime, he came home after battling the boss and office politics, promptly changed into his grubby garden clothes, and proceeded to attack the rose predators. You could almost hear him scolding the beasts and applauding the gorgeous blooms.

All five hundred rose bushes received equal attention as he cycled through them each week, two hours a day, a task my father relished. Despite my early willingness to assist, he later deemed my work inferior and cut me out, pursuing his private thoughts about his cherished blossoms.

The rose-growing season allowed my mother a breath of emancipation with her husband busy elsewhere. Dinners ran late, and the kitchen clean-up became more demanding for me. How she evaded the messes in favor of her bridge group and engaged in solitary drinking or booze-it-up with her brother, Fr. Pius, on his frequent visits remained a mystery. Still, the household hummed a different tune during my late adolescent summers, easing my allergies, especially after Dad cut down the massive cottonwood trees on the edge of the driveway.

The day of my eighteenth birthday felt perfect: radiant sunshine after thunderstorms the previous night; Dad chipper after his two-hour cultivation stint; Mom sober for an entire week. Declaring with a smile that she was "on the wagon," she prepared an abundant feast of roast beef, mashed potatoes, homegrown peas, Waldorf salad, and, my favorite, lemon meringue pie. Feeling expansive, Dad offered me a glass of champagne to honor the birthday girl. To add to the festivities, Dad's three much-loved sisters showed up, bringing homemade bread, pies, and some garden-fresh strawberries.

When the time came for the birthday party corsages, Dad returned from the back garden, his arms embracing a damp newspaper loaded with exquisite roses for his ladies, all seven of us. Staking his claim on the kitchen countertop and pushing us out of the way with his elbow, Dad laid out the roses in neat piles. Even Sharon got her pick of colors.

He sorted flowers by color and size, fastening two or three flowers and barely opening buds onto a crinkly white net, then attaching the rose stem to the netting, he fitted each stem into a miniature water bottle to preserve their freshness. I chose yellow to match my new dress. Of course, Mother had the most gorgeous corsage: a stunning red and white arrangement that highlighted her lovely black hair, leading the aunties to sigh with pleasure.

Three years my junior, Marilyn held her own as the family artist, creating a festive dining room table, arranging flowers, and giving advice on the bathroom wallpaper. Her apparent disregard for parental disapproval seemed to insulate her from their demands. Somehow, she managed to get around our mother's sudden physical attacks and constant nagging about cleaning up paint stains and the pile of dirty clothes.

Dad relaxed with Cappa, Madge, and Ruby, his stalwart sisters who adored their successful brother while sometimes pitying him for putting up with his wife's drunken outbursts. He stayed cheerful, chucking daughters under the chin and putting a protective arm around Mom. I wish this version of my father could prevail forever.

CHAPTER FOURTEEN

Making the Grade

"W hen are you going to get serious about college plans for next year?"

I just shrugged. I felt little enthusiasm to take on college at still another despised Catholic school.

"Ok, Nanette, I'll make a call, and we'll get you moving."

"Moving where?" I asked.

"Getting you into the same school I attended for several years—Northwestern University."

"I can't believe it. Fat chance I could do well in that competition."

But Dad assured me I could do it if I studied harder.

Dad contacted his friend in the registrar's office to smooth my way into that prestigious college.

"I want to provide you with a first-rate education—even if you don't deserve it."

I can't be sure if he referred to my grades, character, or general assessment of my "too-many academic weaknesses," especially in math. Still, I had a grade record that hovered around 95 percent, not perfect and compromised because they came from a Catholic girl's school. Thankfully, the university accepted my academic record.

My co-ed experience during the first college quarter proved to be more than I could handle. Distractions abounded; there was the sorority rush and my initiation into a father-sanctioned Greek house. After four years of dour nuns and a single-gender high school, I encountered a campus full of handsome boys who provided endless dating opportunities. Dreary train commutes from home to school and unspeakable amounts of homework undermined my resolve to "do better." Mountains of home duties and conflicts with parents didn't help the situation. Such disruptions thwarted my best efforts to take Dad's advice and "get serious about school." I felt especially infuriated that my father refused permission for me to live on campus so that I could be a regular college student.

"You're not mature enough," he said, shaking his head.

"So, who's mature?" I retorted. "And what is it anyway?"

Getting only silence, I skipped through the first year, spending most of my time dating cute fraternity boys, or "wolves," as Mom called them. I took every opportunity to hang out in Chicago's musical nightclubs with fabulous jazz performers, develop sorority friends, read novels, and barely kept a B average in required classes.

My father soon recognized he had lost considerable negotiating power. Taking the winter dawn commuter train for eight a.m. lectures and a late return after a long day of classes and library work meant I missed supper *and* housework. I also had less tolerance for his games that once terrorized me. Mom came to my side of the issue.

"Van, she's no help at all around the house," she said. "What's the point of having Nanette live at home if I have to hire all this help, anyway?"

Finally, Dad came up with a plan. I was offered a shiny black Chrysler convertible with red leather seats in exchange for the growing list of housework duties that further cut into my studies and social time. Not such a good deal, after all, but, of course, I took it. Distractions multiplied. I doubt any of us won that round.

Year two began inauspiciously enough. Dad told me my grades needed to improve, or these were my final days of college.

"Imagine, Nanette," he warned, "a 'C' average in Spanish after all that Latin and Spanish study at Marywood! If the university doesn't work out, you can learn some good clerical skills, and I'll help you find a job."

It would never happen, I muttered to myself. I'd run away first. I'd watched Mom make drinks for years; nothing to it. I could always be a bartender on Howard Street.

"You can always make a living as a prostitute, no big deal," whispered a very small, inside voice from one of the Church-condemned books I enjoyed reading. "Anything is better than housework or sitting on your ass, serving some executive like your father."

Finally, Dad conceded on the housing issue only because he was tired of my badgering. I felt lucky because Mom put in a good word for me. Sharon acted happy that I could be a *real* college student, and she may have talked to him about my living in the dorm.

"You can live on campus, but no nonsense," said Dad, his brow stern. "You're going to follow all the rules and get better grades."

"Sure, Dad, no problem."

I applied myself, and studying became a commitment. I moved into a room of my own in the sorority annex where all the students were juniors or seniors and "mature." One gorgeous, long-legged sorority sister insisted she was married, secretly, of course, and slipped away each weekend for a rendezvous—with an invisible husband whom no one ever met.

I found a job at the university library, a few blocks from my new digs, and stopped playing the crazy dating game. I developed new friends, and life picked up speed on a different track. During that first term of living away from home, I finished exams with a flourish. After a few weeks of driving the Chrysler around campus in exchange for weekend home duties, I declined the car and enjoyed leisurely strolls around the tree-lined campus. My life felt strangely sane. I began to be at ease with myself and the world.

Still, I had rebellious holdovers and suffered the consequences. I violated the house curfew of 2:00 a.m. sharp on Saturdays—well, I was only a little late at 2:40 a.m.—and was placed on a strict regimen. House arrest required I return *every* evening by 8:00 p.m. Dad's laughter reinforced what I considered excessive punishment.

"I couldn't have wished it on a more deserving person," he said. "You'll have to learn your lesson about following the rules."

While I failed to appreciate my father's twisted humor at the time, the setback proved useful for tightening my lax school discipline. My available study time was significantly extended, with nothing to do after 8:00 p.m.

I finally felt mature.

CHAPTER FIFTEEN

Violated

The winter of that second year proved to be the hardest yet. The week before tests, I spent all-nighters writing endless term papers, catching up with the 200-pages-a-day reading assignments and smacked into the worst: all-essay exams that bent my overwrought brain into bizarre shapes. Mom laughed when I told her how exhausted I was from the term.

"No rest for the wicked," she pronounced. "Don't worry, Dear. Once you're home for the break, you can catch up. Now, don't get caught up with parties and outings. Take a week and get yourself together. I know how much you need your rest."

When my mother was sober, she was the best!

"OK, Mom," I replied. "No skiing, music, or parties, even if it is Spring Break. I promise I'll stop my frantic running around and spend time with the family. I could use a bit of relaxation after the last term."

Exams finished, I gathered clothes and books, dashed to the train station, caught the Northshore's slow afternoon commuter to Wilmette, then walked head down, against Lake Michigan's bitter mid-March wind, the three blocks to a welcoming home. Everyone was so happy to see me; it was a delightful surprise. I could hardly believe it: absence did make the heart grow fonder.

Sleep. I needed sleep. The bedroom beckoned with darkened shades covering the last vestiges of bleak afternoon light. Even food repelled me; once deliciously familiar, the smells nauseated me. Soon I was carried into a world of enveloping silence.

A phone jangled in my ear. I couldn't have been sleeping for more than an hour. Picking up the phone, I heard the familiar voice of Robert, my Brooklyn pal I met at a party. I playfully called him "Butch," although he wasn't fond of the nickname. Though hardly my heartthrob, he could be funny at times.

"Go away, Butch. I've just finished exams and need to rest for a while."

I suppose I liked Butch because he was on my father's hit list: Jewish, working class, prone to ungrammatical English, and heavy set—a fullback on his university football team weighing in at 230 pounds. My father insisted he even grunted when he talked.

"Hey, I've gotcha a great surprise," Butch persisted. "You don't want to miss it."

"I don't care right now. I can't stir myself out of this bed. This quarter has been a horrible term, with too many classes. Call me tomorrow."

"Can't do that. Have to work at my uncle's used car lot. Aw, come on, that's what I always love 'bout you. You're always ready for a good time—you're the life of the party! Youse ready for anything!"

"Butch, I'm telling you I'm tired, exhausted, finished!"

"OK, honeybun, you sleep. I'm downtown now. It'll take me an hour or so before I make it to your house. Just throw on a skirt and sweater. Promise you, promise you, you're gonna love this surprise."

"All right," I mumbled to avoid the urgent voice.

Later, when Butch picked me up, he was all smiles, humming his favorite ditty.

"Gonna Take a Sentimental Journey."

"What! a new Buick?" I asked.

"Yeah, my uncle's gift for helping him out over the holidays. He's the chief sales guy at the GM dealership, the big 'un on the South Side."

Once seated, I promptly dozed off until Butch pulled up to the curb.

"What's this, Butch?" I said sleepily as I sat up straighter. "It looks like an abandoned building."

"No way, my cousin has been busy remodeling this older hotel. You'll love it. We'll check in with him for a quick minute."

Oh dear, I thought to myself. "This looks like a drag—visiting his family, who, Butch says, detests me. His Aunt Miriam told him, "stay away from the goyim." So, what was he doing dating me?

I stumbled behind him, walking down a long, dark hallway to the last door on the right, which Butch threw open with a flourish.

"Wait here 'til I find my cousin and then what you've been waiting for: the big surprise."

I entered a nearly deserted room, except for a filthy mattress sliding awry off an old metal bed. No curtains, chairs, tables, paintings, or even blankets. Mom would have laughed and said, "What a dump!"

This event was no ordinary date but a set-up. Once Butch turned the key in the lock, his intentions were clear, his face a mask, his demeanor menacing.

The 19-year-old girl I once was proved ill-prepared to cope with a sexual assault, despite the lurid narratives in True Crime magazines she enjoyed for leisure-time reading. These stories depicted willing victims swooning with ecstasy as their attackers took them by force.

Who was this guy, anyway, tearing her clothes, slapping her face, punching her soft body? Who was this young woman trying to defend herself against the bulk of a well-muscled attacker? How could she prevent the malicious deception, the ferocious anger, the shocking violence of someone who appeared to want her dead?

The sharpened knife at her neck was overkill, but it achieved the attacker's objective: submission. The girl began crying, praying, pleading for mercy. Like a wounded animal, she stopped defending herself and whimpered: "please, don't hurt me."

Once the assailant subdued her, he seemed in a hurry to complete the business. His aim was power, not murder. But it took decades for the girl to understand what happened that cold, dark day in March 1950.

Nauseated, nearly unconscious from terror, and shivering uncontrollably, I fumbled for my torn undergarments and wrapped the ripped sweater around me. I pulled my coat tight and prayed for survival. Butch pushed me out the bedroom door, down the dark hallway with a weighty arm on my shoulder, and directed me to the outside door. Once in the car, I huddled against the door, asking God to deliver me from this shameful episode.

Butch returned to his mister-nice-guy-Dr. Jekyll persona, after his wicked performance as monster Mr. Hyde. He cracked jokes, told stories about his relations, recounted his football victories from last season, and turned up his favorite swing band on the new car radio, repeatedly thumping the steering wheel in bursts of delight. At last, he lurched around the corner to drop me off in front of my house.

"So long, Nanette, I'll give ya' a call tomorrow, and let's boogie somewhere downtown. A tremendous little jazz band just came to the Blue Note."

Aghast, I slammed the car door and dashed to the house before Butch changed his mind and came after me again. Where was his remorse? His sense of doing wrong? Making amends? Any sign that he registered my shock, my panic, my horror? Nothing. A blank.

I slipped inside, double-locked the front door, and looked around. No one home, thank God. I promptly got into the shower. I felt dead inside, emptied of myself: feelings, hopes, loves, future, everything now vacant. Not a soul could share my dreadful experience. It would be my fault, anyway. I could hear my accusatory father castigating me for running around with those "low-life fellows."

"You get what you deserve."

* * *

The spring term went on without me. I did not, could not talk to anyone, especially family members. Anger, depression, and guilt lashed through me for weeks, eventually making me sick. I developed a severe cold and laryngitis.

"Butch keeps calling," Mom told me. "He sounds pretty insistent. Why not call him back?"

Every mention of Butch produced a new round of nausea and despair.

"Watch out for the wolves!" My mother always warned me. She meant the kind of guys who stand on the corner, whistling at the pretty girls going by. She never imagined a friend seriously injuring another friend. Date rape existed outside her mental orbit entirely. Her ignorance made it impossible for me to share my horrifying experience.

As for my sisters, I swore myself to secrecy. I planned never to let them know I had been violated, lest they even considered the possibility that such a horror could happen to them: dear pure-hearted Sharon, barely 14 years old. What a misfortune to have a polluted sister forever tainted by a vicious rape.

A final reason I remained silent involved the terror of speaking about the atrocity. Silence weighed heavy, but talking about it brought up countless fears of reliving the degradation again. I kept this silence until the seventh year of my marriage, finally confiding in my loving, supportive husband.

I decided not to return to school, terrified of being injured again. I was even afraid of going outside: me, the big outdoor girl! Instead of calling and letting Butch know how bitterly angry I was, I wrote him a brief letter and sent it to his college address. I had just finished reading Nathaniel Hawthorne's, *The Scarlet Letter* and decided to have Butch answer for his sin in highly dramatic and spiritual terms.

Dear Butch,

You have seriously demeaned yourself and me. You are unworthy of the trust everyone has placed in you, including your parents, brother, sister, University, football team, and, of course, me. I consider you the lowest worm of a human being, but rather than seeing you dead, I curse you.

I curse your birth, childhood, present, future, and even existence. You will never know a moment of peace with the curse I have laid on you to the seventh generation. You will live a miserable life and die a failure without hope or redemption.

Sincerely,

Nanette

Butch's efforts to turn matters around just fueled my anger. On a final phone call, I repeated my curse.

"Never darken my door again," I added, using my mother's familiar expression. "You are a hopelessly evil man."

"I ain't done nothin' wrong," came his limp response.

A week later, Butch sent me a Catholic Bible with the inscription: "Please forgive me."

I tore the sheet out, cut it into tiny bits, and ground it in the garbage disposal.

*   *   *

Later, after months of reflection, I wrote in my journal using the "you" form to create distance from the painful event.

You told yourself that you can't have been the only person humiliated, tortured, and raped by a buddy, just out for fun, a good time—a movie and popcorn date, a walk in the park.

Did you not expect to be violated, or did you, as everyone must have whispered, "bring it on yourself?" A little too free with the laughter, the buddy-boy system with boyfriends, the revealing clothes, the come-hither look of the flirtatious female. They always say that, don't they? It has to be your fault.

Who told you that you're not the only one to have this horrific experience? How would you know? As far as you're concerned, you're the only one who's ever been degraded, isolated, lost, anguished, filled with self-loathing; so much grieving and, oh so heartbroken; just broken.

What happened? Wrong place, wrong time, wrong guy, wrong, wrong, wrong. You wanted to talk with someone so much and share the sadness and distress. But all of us—silenced by fear.

* * *

Month followed month with what I believed was a pregnancy. After all, I had all the symptoms, the same symptoms my mother had when she was pregnant with little brother Davey when I was eleven: no menstrual period, morning nausea, belly swelling, tender nipples, and crippling fatigue.

I confronted a second major hurdle: what to do about this? Terrified of rejection but desperate to find an ally, I called a college buddy, Gary, who was in my speech class. Although my age of 19, he always seemed so young, so innocent, one of eight children from a Philadelphia suburb. Maybe, I could confide in him.

I spilled out my tragic story, and I was right. I found a sympathetic ear, one who listened without judging.

Together we plotted our course, looking at alternatives. Gary thought it would be fun to hop on a ship to South America, have the baby, and never return home. No sin involved, except stealing money from our parents to carry out the daring journey. Of course, we never considered melting into the greater Chicago area or a nearby city, working and paying for the baby. Only a dramatic exit would do. But I wavered.

"Gary, there must be a better way. I can't do this to my family. I also know I could never, ever tell them. Simply disappearing would be a nightmare for them and my sisters and brother. Why would I do this to people I love?"

The final solution: find an abortion doctor to add to my total shame and commit another mortal sin. I would never be forgiven, anyway. So, why not go through with it and wipe out evidence of my iniquities?

We located a doctor in Northside Chicago who practically advertised his specialty in the Yellow Pages, though subtle too—"let me handle your most intimate problems—and mistakes." We looked for more information and found it from one of the local bartenders in the neighborhood.

"Dr. Dread operates out of his apartment," he told us. "A fairly classy brick building two blocks off the main drag. Look for a red Pontiac at the curb."

Once on the brittle, cold table, the doctor pushed and probed.

"No anesthetic here, I'm afraid," he said. "Too dangerous. It helps if you relax."

He was brusque, giving no small talk, and lacked any bedside manner to ease a terrified patient as he stuffed a rag in my mouth to muffle my shrieks. I couldn't speak for the pain because of the cloth. He continued to palpate my abdomen.

"Oh my God," I thought. "I feel as though I am being raped all over again."

Then, he suddenly stopped, took a careful look at my desolate face, and said,

"No pregnancy here. You'd better make an appointment with your regular doctor to ensure you haven't got a medical problem."

Jumping off the examining table, I paid the doctor a small fortune of $125 and lunged at the nearest bar for a frothy pink lady and a greasy hamburger with my best buddy, Gary.

I knew in my heart that this experience was my first look at the gargoyle of mental illness: the transformation of an ordinary, decent person, my friend Butch, into an unconscious, violent offender, a maddened monster. Why me? This question lingered for years.

Butch took on the curse, as I learned from his buddies who attended the same school. First, he dropped out of the football team, and without a football scholarship to pay the tuition, left the university a term later. Failing miserably at the full-time job in his uncle's car dealership, Butch wasn't fun anymore -- no more jokes, and stories, all gone. I learned from his cousin he often appeared dejected and despondent. I later learned that his life continued on a downward spiral: failed marriages, alcoholism, and bankruptcy.

Both parents rallied during my "confinement," knowing something deplorable had happened to me. Amazingly, they allowed me to express sadness, deep moodiness, and even bizarre behavior, hoping it would pass. They never said a disparaging word. No one asked me to do housework. I never volunteered. I wondered if they knew something.

Once I left the Chicago area, I embraced a new life in Minneapolis— on Dad's suggestion since he had contacts there. Beyond doubt, he realized I wanted "out" of the family, my hometown, and my present school.

I seized the opportunity to fashion a self-fulfilling existence. I tackled school at the University of Minnesota, met my future husband, Jim, learned to live independently, and opened my heart to life on new terms. Only after these changes could I let go of the anger, guilt, and oppression. What remained? A deep caution: find a rescuer; do not step outside the bounds; stay invisible.

Part Two

CHAPTER SIXTEEN

Leaving Home

Marilyn and I were absentee sisters for much of Sharon's growing up. After all, I moved away, and Marilyn was busy with art. Marilyn discovered her artistic gift at an early age. She regularly took the train to the Chicago Art Institute for lessons twice a week, feverishly working in her bedroom to complete art lessons. My mother's big gripe was how much the art lessons cost. But I overheard Dad's rejoinder to Mom.

"I think Marilyn has real talent," he said. "I spoke with her art teacher, and he's quite impressed with her progress. She loves this work; that's reason enough to pay for lessons."

He could finally relax about Marilyn having problems at New Trier. She was doing much better than he expected at the public school and insisted, over our mother's objections, that Sharon should also avoid the Catholic school. Besides, he persisted:

"I'm sick and tired of paying for all that tuition. I've heard enough griping about "being at the wrong school. "Let's not forget that Nanette hated Marywood and even refused to attend her graduation ceremony." It seems my travails at Marywood rescued Marilyn and Sharon from a similar fate.

When I occasionally talked to Sharon on the phone while attending the University of Minnesota, she moaned about "not dating yet," comparing her open weekends to my former lavish dating activities.

"Maybe I'm too young, or probably, I never will find a boyfriend in this high school."

It seemed to temporarily assuage her worries when I reassured her that she was only 15 and she had plenty of time to date. I suspect Sharon continued to lament her less-than-trendy lifestyle because she felt invisible in a highly competitive high school.

After the rape episode, Sharon overheard me shouting and cursing Butch on the phone. It was the last anyone ever heard from him, especially after I sent him the fearful curse through the mail. I stayed closed-mouthed about the entire tragedy. But when she kept asking what was wrong, I yelled out, "He injured my soul, and I cursed the bastard into eternity!" Perhaps that was more dramatic than necessary in light of Sharon's tender age.

Following Sharon's lead, I started writing in one of Dad's empty journals. It seemed to help. Strangely, I never had any guilt about condemning Butch. His damnation poured out of me naturally and never provoked regret.

June, three months after the worst experience of my life, I hitched a ride with two student pals, Gary and Steve, all three of us planning to sign up at the University of Minnesota. Just as my father had rigged up my entrance into Northwestern University, he figured out my next move, determining that a change of scene would do me good. Against Mom's alarming outcries, Dad convinced her he would pay for a visit, giving her a chance to look over my progress. The journaling gave me the strength to think about getting out of that town and starting a new life.

When Mom showed up for her maternal oversight, I snarled up any attempt at appropriately entertaining my guest. Having no familiarity with the downtown, I erroneously took her to a gay bar featuring the "finest queens in the north." Initially, my mother just stared at these elaborately costumed men, then protested about their "sinning," and finally, sitting back, laughed through the entire show. A cheap meal at the diner was the price for my awkward choice of entertainment that lacked a dinner menu.

I was happy for the first time in months, away from my oppressive environment, thrilled to be leaving my despoiled self behind. My father may have had other rationales for letting me go: a more serene household, his promise to Mom she could have plenty of cleaning women and laundry service once I wasn't available, and maybe his fingers were crossed that I'd meet the right man. Of course, the right man would have a high-paying job, relieving dad of the financial burden of supporting me.

When I brought home scholarly Jim, just completing his doctoral studies, Dad must have been puzzled. This guy was unlike all those "losers" who used to trail in and out of the house. True to form, Dad could not leave it alone, but Jim proved a worthy adversary for his challenges.

"I can't believe you're taking a government job instead of aiming for college administration. There's no money in government work, no point in traipsing off to Washington, D.C., and parts unknown. And you say you eventually want to teach college? Those who can't do, teach," Dad mocked.

Undeterred, Jim met every argument with systematic reasoning. Although his political forte was academic, his daily reading of *The New York Times* provided a steady flow of economic and political facts that my father admired. Once he tacitly accepted Jim, Dad gloated over his brilliant, soon-to-be son-in-law, even if he "would never make a penny."

My mother embarrassed me even more, aggressively attacking Jim because he wasn't Catholic and, at 11 years my senior, certainly too old for me.

"You have to promise you will raise your children Catholic."

After a few drinks, she grumbled to no one in particular: "What's Nanette doing not marrying one of the nice boys from St. Joseph's parish?"

"You're entirely too old for her. Imagine my young, beautiful daughter marrying such an older man. You're nearly my age!"

I knew Mom had a thing about age, constantly chopping a few years off her own when she could. But what really grated on her was that my future, always polite, fiancé did not drink: no beer, wine, or cocktails, no alcohol at all. My decision to marry a non-drinking man was deliberate. I had no wish to repeat the chaos of my growing-up years.

The house was in an uproar, getting ready for the big day. We yearned for a small wedding with a few friends. Mom and Dad demanded the works: Mom because she wanted to show off, Dad because he wanted to get even.

"After all, I've paid for wedding gifts for all those employees' kids," he said. "Now it's my turn."

It was OK with Jim, he was willing to accommodate his future in-laws' demands, but I thought it was all too materialistic—and stupid.

Mom's nightly tangents and Dad's confrontational exchanges spurred my wish to get this wedding over with—fast. I told Jim, "let's get this wedding on the road so we can start our married life free from this harassment." But wedding plans dragged on.

From March to September, my mother, the wedding planner, played out her grand designer role: guest lists, invitations, dinner favors, venue, trousseau, bridal parties, celebrant, and meal choices. She even broadcasted her expansive plans for our honeymoon to everyone she knew. Aside from visiting her brother and sister-in-law, my Uncle Pat, and Aunt Florence in an upscale Detroit suburb, we pursued our wishes for post-wedding travels at a Canadian fishing resort. We opted for simple.

Unaided by either Jim or me, Mother could not be persuaded from her ceremonial role. When I expressed my lack of interest, Mom lassoed my delighted sisters, Sharon and Marilyn, as bridesmaids, requiring more shopping for the perfect outfits.

I threw my hands up: this wasn't my wedding at all. Mom's version of a *Ladies Home Journal* wedding seemed atrocious. I recall shopping with Sharon and Mom, seeking the ideal wedding dress and trousseau, which took me away from my real estate job. I resented all the time I had to take off from work, needing as much money as possible to buy our first car. Jim's summer insurance job could only pay for the honeymoon and first month's rent for our new, furnished apartment.

Mom especially crowed over the wedding dress: straps/strapless, long/mid-length; lacy/plain; silk/organdy. I chose plain; Mom picked out only extravagant. After feuding for days, we settled on organza material, a mid-length skirt, a simple strapless bodice, and a lacy jacket. I wore this ensemble nightly on our destination cruise to Japan two years later, heading for Jim's new job, officially a "naval intelligence officer," but an undercover agent, in reality.

Jim played out the nice-guy role to the hilt. Detecting that our father had little interest in teaching Sharon how to drive, he asked Dad's permission to take over Sharon's driving lessons. Another coup! Dad was only too happy to discontinue the annoying lessons. Sharon had the same experience learning to drive a car I had with Dad's outbursts. I imagine him saying typical Dad remarks:

"Sharon, for God's sake, hit the brake." Or "you're the worst driver I've ever seen!" And worse, "only a lunatic would have made that left-hand turn."

Jim was invariably supportive. Sharon found him a calm and reassuring coach, which she often mentioned.

Jim told her. "You're a very good driver, and don't worry about making a few mistakes. You know what you're doing."

A significant feature of a Catholic wedding involved two months of attending a religious workshop, a premarital spiritual program. My mother found this arrangement the second-best solution to the religious issue since Jim refused to convert to Catholicism. On Mom's insistence, we borrowed the family car, driving into the city for regular classes "to make sure we would raise the children Catholic."

Jim chaffed under the pre-Vatican doctrines but said little. I was outraged when the priest told the class, "Women must learn obedience, my daughters, as your husband governs you." Keeping silent, I squirmed miserably in the pew. I had no intention of turning over my life to any man. I soon learned that the military-type structure of Jim's work, multiple pregnancies, lack of income, social isolation, and the burden of housework kept me very dependent.

My life seemed a bundle of contradictions during this wedding preparation. Embedded in orthodox theology for part of the week, I argued about economics with Dad the rest of the time. Fruitless arguments, it turned out, my dad holding tight to capitalism, and me, waving the flag for Marxism or other anti-capitalist views. Sharon rolled her eyes at our weird arguments with unpronounceable words.

I felt truly changed: I was much quieter and more thoughtful, not the flighty girl I had been. This ordeal of staying with my parents until Jim and I were safely married wore my patience thin. The most irritating part was Mom and Dad watching their nightly television programs. What an abomination. I turned to Sharon.

"Can you believe it? Mom and Dad roared with laughter at 'I Love Lucy' and ate in the living room on television trays. Mom doesn't even cook anymore; she buys those dreadful TV dinners."

I vowed then I would learn to be a good cook, and never stoop to shortcuts, an abandoned promise once I started graduate school with a house full of ever-hungry children.

*   *   *

The wedding day dawned. Dad walked me down the aisle to Father Hugh O'Flaherty, Mom's pick. We celebrated the mass, and the reception duly followed at a local hall. Here, I confronted a roomful of virtual strangers, my parents' friends and neighbors, and my father's inner circle at work.

As Jim and I were preparing to leave the reception, I overheard Mom telling Sharon that the wedding "was a whopping success!"

"They got away with a lot of loot! Nanette's gifts will fill the entire backseat of the Ford, the car they bought with the money she earned working for the real estate office. She and Jim will do fine in their new apartment in Washington D.C."

Mom seemed to forget how much I wanted out of that job. At one point, I told Sharon to avoid secretarial work, "a dreadful occupation."

I always complained about my nemesis, dragon-lady boss, Miss Needham, who showed up at the reception and acted quite decent. She charmed Dad with her esoteric knowledge of the real estate market.

At the reception, Sharon told me she felt more grown up since the wedding where she served as my bridesmaid. She spoke of being resolute about college coming up in two years, confiding that she planned to be a different person than the "fly-on-the-wall" that Mom called her. I applauded her efforts to make something of herself.

As we joyfully prepared to launch our new life after the festivities, my father drew me aside in our living room, sternly warning: "You made your bed; now you lie in it." I stared at him, horrified. What a strange send-off—for any daughter! I determined then that I would make this marriage work, whatever it took.

Our married life was off to a good start, and with little Kathy now 11 months old, we began elaborate preparations for Jim's overseas assignment. Getting ready for a two-year stint in Asia required a final visit home. The folks found it inexplicable that we'd be going to Japan, our former enemy in WWII, and after that, an even more ends of the earth place, the Philippine Islands. Neither country felt safe to them, especially not a defeated nation. Mom's complaints mainly focused on losing touch with the new baby.

"Little Kathy needs her Grandma. It's my first grandchild. I'm so thrilled. Now I can wear that cute grandma charm bracelet your Dad bought me at the jewelry store." But when she rattled her new acquisition in front of Kathy, the baby let out a howl that ended the discussion.

When she inquired about why we had to go to Asia for such a long time, I shrugged my shoulders.

"It's part of his job, Mom." As non-overseas travelers in that period, my parents found any excursion that took them out of their comfort zone to be out of the question. There I was, gloating over my grand escape, leaving Sharon barren of even my remote presence.

While my family and I traveled and absorbed new cultures, Sharon finished high school and sought the more secure environment of a women's Catholic college, St. Theresa's College, which welcomed the daughters of managers, promising to give them a good education but also career training. Even without Mom's prompting, Dad considered Catholic training superior to secular colleges. The smaller print read: "...in the event your husband dies or is disabled."

"Catholic education offers the biggest bang for the buck because it instills social values and discipline, as well as having smaller classes and more dedicated faculty," he said. "You can't get all that at the University of Illinois, Marilyn's last school."

It turns out Sharon could ham it up, Mom said in a letter. Involved in theater, clubs, and making straight As, Sharon starred in her freshman-year school play, "The Importance of Being Ernest." I only remember the monstrous defeat of being fired from the lead role in my senior high school class play because I continuously showed up late for rehearsals.

Sharon was dating the "dreamiest boy," Matt, another of Mom's letters gushed.

"He attends the men's Catholic school across the river." I could feel Mom's excitement rising as she detailed Sam's background. "His dad is a lawyer from a well-to-do, prominent Catholic family."

Both parents were relieved that Sharon's college had strict rules about curfew and alcohol. As far as I knew, Sharon never defied them.

Then came the crushing letter about Sam not responding to Sharon's letters after he graduated and went on to graduate school. Mom reported that Sharon had been miserable and not open to her attempts to comfort her. Mom probably told Sharon: "First loves don't always turn out. Buck up, lots more boys for you once you graduate."

Our folks were elated with Sharon's achievements and minimized the loss of her boyfriend. Her successes were often the focus of mom's bi-weekly letters.

"Sharon's a model student who traveled with us to Hawaii last year. Next year, she plans to study in Grenoble, France, as a language major. Dad thinks she's a great candidate to be a foreign language teacher." It seemed a far-fetched claim, considering Dad's antipathy to teaching as a lesser occupation.

Dad always pointed out the importance of self-sufficiency, although I'm not confident my sisters received that message. Like the Catholic college brochure, which focused on careers, Dad reminded me, "it's important to think about a livelihood." For my father, it was only in case my husband died.

I often wondered about Sharon. I thought that she wanted to prove herself in a career after graduation and show the world she was more intelligent than some people thought. She had already demonstrated to family, college faculty, and the body of college students that she was no longer a fly on the wall.

In the meantime, I proceeded to show off my maternity powers, having one baby after another: three daughters, Kathy, Susie, and Liddy followed by Timmy and Mikey, and six years later, our sweet Patti, named after my cousin, Patricia, who died young in an airplane crash.

This family of mine was a large order, but it worked sublimely well until our family hit a major snag with our fifth child.

CHAPTER SEVENTEEN

Faith by Deception

"We'd love to see the children this summer, but your Dad is too busy with work and can't visit, and I know you're tied up in a legislative campaign with Jim and could use some help," Mom said on a phone call.

She was right. Since Jim decided to run for state legislator from our district, we'd worked day and night, knocking on doors and giving talks in homes, churches, and community centers. Jim was doing most of the campaigning, but his campaign manager recruited me to do more coffee klatches in voters' homes. It all seemed preposterous. How could I ever do more with five small children?

But can I count on Mom? She sounded very lucid on the phone, but her mood changes, and she's off to the races with her martini habit. I think I'll forget it for now.

But my mother kept calling, imploring me to send the three little girls. Timmy, age six, and Mikey, age two, my two small ones, would be my responsibility. She promised the girls Grandma and Grandpa would offer lots of outdoor, healthy California air, go to nearby sandy beaches, and take them for picnics every weekend. The offer seemed ideal, especially in light of the increased pressure I was getting from Jim's campaign manager to meet and greet the voters. The following story depicts many details furnished years later by my older daughters, especially Susan, who recalled every particular.

* * *

Three small girls huddled closely together on the cold bench on a raw spring day in 1964. They were waiting for their special gift, Catholic baptism. Grandma told them it was exceptional, because the Monsignor himself would be here in Grandma and Grandpa's house to administer the Holy Sacrament. Grandma still wasn't out of bed to dress them for this celebratory occasion. The three home-bound children had yet to have a picnic, a beach trip, or even an outing. Instead, they daily faced the rigors of memorizing the Catholic catechism, so unlike the easy Biblical stories recited in their weekly Presbyterian Sunday school.

The oldest girl, Kathy, age 11, hushed the youngest one, Liddy, who found the entire situation dismal at seven years old. "Where's Mommy and Daddy?" she sobbed. Susie took aim at her runny nose, tissue in hand, but Liddy dodged her and let out an angry howl in the face of this persecution.

Nine-year-old Sue, the peacemaker, adept in mollifying her little sister, said.

"Okay, Honey. Here comes Grandpa now, and he's "madder than a hatter," as Mommy says. "Let's all smile and be happy. "Hi, Grandpa," the three dutifully called out.

"Get in here and get yourselves dressed. Grandma isn't feeling well, and Monsignor Greeley is due here in half an hour. I've got the space set up for the baptism. You girls will have to dress yourselves. Hurry it up!"

He turned abruptly and dashed to the front door. "Goddamn it, why does Alice have to have a hangover today," the grandfather muttered.

"Sweet Sue," her Daddy called her. Accustomed to caring for her younger, difficult brother, Mikey, Sue gently wiped Liddy's nose and slipped the white baptismal dress over her head. Little Liddy smiled. The day was beginning to come together, even if the lovely new frocks were on still-to-be-bathed children.

The Monsignor's arrival signaled the grandmother's hastily assembled morning routine. Just a few personal details and arrangements, and within minutes, she swept into the expansive living room where the Monsignor and his two attendants stood waiting. The children couldn't help but notice Grandma's blouse spilling over her skirt and her elegant silk stocking cascading down one leg.

"Good morning, Mrs. Trexler. How are you doing?"

"Perfect," she exclaimed, extending a trembling hand to the dignitary. "Hello, Monsignor Greeley. This is an honor officiating at the baptism of my three granddaughters from Minnesota. Van will be bringing them in shortly. We can start in a few minutes."

"Are the godparents ready?" The Monsignor asked.

"Yes indeed," the Grandmother said. "I have a husband and wife for each child serving as godparents. We also have some parish friends joining us as witnesses. Here they are now. Van is answering the door even as we speak. One more thing: the girls' parents couldn't make it today; I'm so sorry. My son-in-law, Dr. Davis, couldn't leave his college administrative job, and my daughter has a severe cold."

She carefully kept silent about the real reason for the parents' absence. Pre-Vatican II treated Grandmother's little white lies as only venial sins, compared to the mortal stakes of unbaptized children. How could she approach Jim, her son-in-law, a staunch Christian Scientist, who would be violently opposed to this underhanded move? And her daughter, a lapsed Catholic, who would never accept baptism by fiat. The Grandmother had to take it upon herself to do the right thing. She alone could save these souls from a fate worse than death: their perpetual existence in Limbo for all eternity.

"Monsignor Greeley, once we've finished with the baptism, we'll adjourn into the dining room for a lovely lunch I've prepared. I don't want to send you and your baptismal team away hungry," she laughed.

Monsignor Greeley was one of Grandmother's favorites; a sweet Irishman, if ever she's seen one. The Monsignor enjoyed his cocktails now and then, at which time they called each other "Pete and Alice." They got along beautifully.

"Very good. Have the children completed their catechism lessons and are ready to fully accept their new identity in the Lord Jesus through Catholic baptism?"

"Yes, Excellency. Van and I have been working with them for a couple of weeks. Our seven-year-old is a bit bull-headed, but she'll be fine. Of course, the older girls find it easier to master the lessons. You know how some kids can be," she giggled.

The Monsignor nodded sagely, having no idea how any kids can be, having had no interaction with children for the past 25 years of his priesthood. Baptism was different, of course. He dealt with souls, not persons, and he aimed to keep his focus clear today.

The Grandmother had quizzed each child the day before.

"Baptism will be the most important day of your life. You must agree to accept this gift of the Holy Spirit. Do you consent to have this sacrament?"

Nine-year-old Sue shivered amid this twisted religious event. As an adult, she told me how she felt during the ordeal.

"Tears came to my eyes. But I wasn't used to crying in front of people, and certainly not Grandma Alice, who hovered over me, her face hard, but smiling her red-lipsticked clown's mouth. 'Oh, yes,' I lied, forcing myself to smile. What did my grandmother think? That I'd say no, in front of her? When I'd never defied a grown-up in my life. 'I want to.' I imagine my sisters told the same lie."

The ceremony commenced. "In the name of the Father, and of the Son, and of the Holy Spirit," Monsignor Greeley intoned, starting the sacred moment with the sign of the cross.

The girls stared mutely as the priest covered each small head with water and the sign of the cross, followed by a sturdy toweling by one of the acolytes. The ritual continued: candles were distributed to grandparents and godparents with promises made by the grandchildren to faithfully follow the commandments and Catholic precepts. Witnesses snapped photos, and at last, the children were pacified.

The baptismal party followed the Grandmother into the dining room for the ceremonial feast: roasted ham, fried chicken, potato salad, green salad, and the Grandmother's favorite: lemon meringue pie. The grandmother's two favorite Irish maids, Patty and Rosy, helped assemble the culinary delights. Those cherished girls, soon gone, would be supplanted by African American staff, newly arrived from Georgia.

The Monsignor smiled benignly as he devoured the splendid refreshments, including cocktail-sized glasses of the finest sour mash bourbon, abundantly supplied by Van to all the guests. The Monsignor's prompting encouraged Alice to make this rash move to prevent heathenism from smashing into the family tree.

"Imagine," he had emphasized, "unbaptized children, their immortal souls forever absent from God's mercy. Unthinkable," he added. He told the grandmother that she had a duty and right to intervene. "In fact," he pontificated, "your soul is lost if you ignore this opportunity to bring these souls into the Catholic fold."

Alice nodded gravely, ignoring the reality of who would pursue the Catholic training and guidance once she returned the grandchildren to their parents.

The newly blessed children, lifted onto the oversize dining room chairs, could now be ignored as the adults returned to their drinking, eating, and private conversations. Kathy and Susie ate contentedly, carefully following their parents' strictures about proper table manners. Little Liddy, squirming miserably, began her soft sobbing that, within minutes, was mixed with coughing and gagging.

Jumping from his seat, the grandfather pulled the limp child into his arms, shouting: "Oh my God, Alice. This child has a fever. Call the doctor immediately!"

Little Liddy suffered in bed for seven days with raging pneumonia, a fever of 105 degrees, and shouts and curses from Van. He told the Grandmother she should never have pulled this stunt without letting the parents know beforehand.

"The children are too young. It's not our charge to push religion. Let their parents take care of the matter. If our son-in-law considers a legal option, he could accuse you of kidnapping the children. After all, little Liddy is still at death's door. And we've never even called their parents to tell them of her serious illness."

"Now, Van, Liddy will be fine. The Monsignor has been over every day this week, blessing her, and yesterday she received Extreme Unction, the sacrament for the dying," she hastened to inform her husband. Poor Van, she thought, how could he understand the mysteries of the Church? His German Protestant background continues to leave him spiritually empty.

"Liddy's sure to survive. Monsignor Pete is a prince whose prayers will pull her through. Now, please, let's calm down."

But the Grandfather would not be calmed. Van had a different view of the Monsignor and his unwelcome intrusion into their lives. Over the last few years, he had observed the prelate's undue influence over his wife, spending more time doing diocesan work and writing large checks for various causes. These financial contributions earned the Monsignor's attention, rewarding Alice with frequent home visits and extended cocktail hours, where his wife gazed with pleasure at his handsome Irish face.

Van remained suspicious about Alice's intense attraction to Irish clergy, whom she claimed looked like her dear Dad, who sorrowfully, she invariably sighed, passed away nearly 50 years ago.

Departure day. A weak, but feverless Liddy, crawled into the car with her two sisters, and they were off to the train station. Neither their parents nor grandparents found it unusual to allow these unattended youngsters to travel alone from the Chicago suburbs to St. Cloud, Minnesota.

"Now, girls," the Grandmother gave her final, prayerful advice. "Pray daily, and make your parents take you to the Catholic Church every Sunday without fail. No other religion will do. Holy Mother Church can only save us through the Blessed Sacraments. You'll be happy to hear that we plan on having Holy

Communion and Confirmation next year. The Monsignor told me he'd be happy to officiate at our nearby St. Joseph's Church."

The three small girls quivered. "Of course, Grandma," they said in subdued voices as they boarded the Chicago Northwest Railroad to their Minnesota home, their flawed faith wavering behind them, ready to float away with the first breeze of the moving train.

CHAPTER EIGHTEEN

The Years of
Living Disastrously

Our second son, Michael, born in 1962, had a difficult start in life. The pediatrician discovered his legs had been twisted in the womb and placed him in leg braces that severely hampered free movement. From six to nearly 18 months old, little Mike would drag his legs with their heavy braces from room to room, postponing both crawling and walking stages. Worse, the brace situation created a cranky, needy child, always demanding to be picked up rather than deal with the discomfort, and sometimes pain, of moving on his own.

Four-year-old Timmy, our family's spoiled darling, had only anger at the birth of another child. Timmy hammered loudly on the closed door when the infant was sleeping in their shared bedroom, kicking and pounding, eventually pushing his small fist through the cheap wood panel. "Mike's awake again, screaming," I moaned. Jim intervened, reluctantly spanking the older brother. Still, Timmy doggedly continued at every opportunity until Jim hung a heavier door and bought miniature boxing gloves for the irate child to pound elsewhere.

His older sister, Sue, ever the kind little mother, took Mike under her care, soothing and quieting his peevish outbursts. The baby squirmed continuously with the weight, the braces pinching, the legs aching. Compared with the four older babies, Mike seemed to need excessive pacifying. The little one got on everyone's nerves with his frequent shrill cries, a condition that persisted long after removing the braces. With Patti's birth in 1968, Sue abandoned care for six-year-old Mike, shifting to the new baby as her special charge. It was as though Mike had dropped out of sight.

I knew Jim felt pity and guilt, his son looking distressed with the steel brackets locking his legs together, forcing them into a straight position. He also felt shame because the boy's legs had been damaged, just as his own had been from polio at 11 months. Never a rational process, Mike became Daddy's special boy, whose every whimper received attention, not merely in childhood but throughout his teens and twenties.

Mike grew up handicapped in multiple ways. The phrase, "don't get him started," required every family member to be on high alert, never to disturb or agitate Mike. It wasn't merely his screaming but also the stunts he would pull: cutting up his shoes to get new ones, throwing the cat on the roof, setting the yard on fire, and by age 12, molesting his baby sister, Patti. Mike's oddities and cruelties separated him from both friends and siblings. Sue remembers how he could be a pest, a nuisance; no one liked him; he sat alone as a small boy at his own birthday parties. More than once, I overheard Jim grumbling about carrying an albatross on his back.

While I tried to treat Mike as a normal child with soothing phrases, "Now, Honey, let's just calm down, it's not a calamity, we can work it out," Jim often interrupted to meet whatever demands Mike made: the father bought the new shoes, he coaxed the cat off the roof, and hosed down the burnt lawn. Anything to "shut him up." When Mike began using drugs, Jim didn't hesitate. Pulling money out of his pocket, he would ask his 17-year-old drug-addled son, who supplied contraband to his buddies, "how much?"

But Mike could be such an affectionate child when he felt loved and protected. I vividly recall his sixth birthday when the family gathered at a local restaurant. Mike wanted a hot dog, only a hot dog. Halfway through his meal, he began choking, a piece of meat lodged in his windpipe. Without a word, I leaped up, grasped the child, turning him upside down, and began pounding on his upper back. His breath returned. We all cheered. Mike covered my face with kisses, "I love you, Mommy. Thanks for saving me." Two months later, Patti was born, and Mike lost his unique place in the family constellation, which seriously impacted his young life.

As young as the first and second grades, Mike remembers how his Dad coddled him. "My Dad always spoiled me, and I got my way, usually against my mother's will. I always wanted to go to the store and get a prize or something. I think he [Dad] knew I had great sensitivity and mood swings as a kid, always laughing and crying in a short period of time, and imbalances in the same moment."

Mike believed his difficulties originated with our family moving from one state to another and one school to another, where he was always the outsider, unable to make friends. Rather than gaining more independence as he developed, he turned to the family, almost totally dependent on his father and older brother, Tim. His later involvement with a Twelve-Step sponsor encouraged him to keep a journal to record his experiences and feelings.

"From the very start, I moved around. Since I was four years old, I remember moving...it was difficult in my family life. Along with all the moving, I went to nine different schools until graduation at eighteen. I had mental, social, and psychological problems, so turned to Dad for a fix."

Once Jim left Washington, D.C., for college teaching, he was a man in a hurry. His first academic career job location to St. Cloud, Minnesota, lasted seven years. The next move to Mt. Pleasant, Michigan, involved another seven years, this time, the family moved twice, once into a small ranch-style house and later into a second, larger home outside town to accommodate our sixth child. This required the children to change schools. Every relocation created a bombardment of symptoms for our at-risk child. Mike only wanted to have a "sense of belonging," so precarious for him as he shifted towns and schools.

"In the third grade, I was in my second school. It was about half a mile through the woods. The new school [after the campus elementary school closed down] was cool. Some of my former classmates went there. I remember a great feeling and sense of belonging. I moved again in the fifth and sixth grades to the third school. My family moved, all eight of us, away from town. It was the most difficult time of my life and the beginning of a nightmare [finding friends]."

Eventually, Mike found a friend, Johnny, whom he met on the school bus, who was even more susceptible than Mike, but for that little guy, it was asthma. Any excitement jarred his system, and he would begin intense coughing. Keeping Johnny safe meant Mike had to quiet down his intensity when they were together; interims I tried to expand for family peace. The boys enjoyed one another's company with sleepovers and multiple meals, and Johnny soon became a family fixture. I encouraged his spending long weekends with Mike and special dinners during the week. Johnny's parents seemed almost overly appreciative of the arrangement. I later discovered Mike's friend could not tolerate his parents, who fought all the time and were only too happy to be relieved of their son's care.

But Johnny's weak lungs could no longer take the Michigan winters or the parents' constant squabbling. Eventually, the boy was institutionalized in Arizona without his parents, and we lost connection. I was concerned that Mike would unravel, but he began spending more time with his older brother, Tim, and his sisters at the small country club. Two miles from our country home, the children could ride their bikes back and forth, spending summer days swimming, playing pool, and meeting new friends.

By the sixth grade, Mike seemed to rally. "I was the teacher's pet. Her husband worked in the political science department at the university where my dad chaired. I did very well, like a hot shot. I was a major kickball star, too. Then a nightmare struck when Dad had to make a career move to Bellingham, Washington."

Mike had his first psychotic episode a year later, in 1974, a period of family upheaval and change. Jim put our beautiful two-acre brick home for sale without informing me. He made the solo decision to take a job offer from Western Washington University in Bellingham, Washington, taking only his older son, Tim, leaving me with Mike, Sue, and Patti, and two coed renters whose monthly payments were keeping Katherine and Liddy at the state university about 80 miles away.

Jim failed to negotiate for the first time in our marriage, cutting me loose to make the best of things. Jim took care of the mortgage, but there was so much more: utilities, food, tuition, home, car maintenance, clothing—the financial demands seemed endless. I took on extra classes and even additional teaching jobs, further cutting into the time I could spend with my children.

While Mike experienced ongoing agony, separated from his father and brother, and weekends, I was hopping on airplanes to teach graduate social work students in Kansas City, the pay enticing enough to work seven days a week. In all likelihood, I was too exhausted to pay attention to the void in our family circle.

For six months, Mike barely endured his Dad's absence. Unknown to me, he had turned his frustration outward against his six-year-old sister, Patti. Sue and I noticed her behavior change, insisting on wearing boy's clothing, especially flannel shirts. "Call me Patrick," she insisted, thrusting out her lower lip and right hip. Our little girl looked even more adorable with her latest act, and we deemed it completely natural, having two older brothers. But we all missed the fact that Patti's not-so-cute gender dysphoria originated from older brother Mike's molestation.

Our marriage near tatters, Jim decided the right thing to do was assemble the entire family and have a vacation in the nation's capital. Jittery Mike would then return with his dad and brother to Washington State. While Mike was elated, their father abandoned the rest of the family. I was still trying to sell the house, requiring strenuous efforts to keep the home in elegant condition, running ragged with overwork, and disengaging from old friends and colleagues with my upside-down lifestyle.

I found my deepest friendships with former interviewees from my Ph.D. dissertation on illegal abortion, completed a year ago. Women who worked underground to identify safe abortion procedures during the stormy days of criminalization revealed hearts of compassion. They buoyed me, gave me confidence, and made me wonder why I thought I needed to stay with a man who had left me. What can I do in small town Bellingham? I can't practice my profession because Jim would be my immediate supervisor. University policy against nepotism ruled unopposed.

"You're right! I can support myself and my kids on my own," I told them, and once the Mt. Pleasant house sold, I decided to take the job offer from Michigan State and buy a home in East Lansing. I needed a life, and like all my children, I needed to establish myself. I was torn emotionally. Jim appeared to have entirely cut himself off from the family, even failing to call me when I was in the hospital for minor surgery. The longer we lived apart, the more acrimonious we behaved toward one another. I was profoundly troubled and unsure whether I had made the right decision about a permanent separation.

I was working late, as usual, on a Friday in my university sociology office, not a soul around, when the phone rang. I usually wouldn't have picked up at 8:00 p.m., but absentmindedly, I took the phone call.

"Hello, I'd like to speak to Nanette Davis," the voice said. The call came from Portland State University, three hours difference in time. Otherwise, no one would have answered that fateful call from the West Coast, as my phone lacked voice mail.

The invitation involved a full-time, tenure-track appointment without an interview, an offer I could not refuse. I hastened to contact the realtor to cancel my contract, with only one day before the East Lansing house would be mine.

With the Mt. Pleasant house sold under us, my university contract canceled, and my children scattered to the winds with friends, I had no choice but to stay in a tiny affordable college dormitory room for six weeks until the end of the school term. In mid-June, Katherine, Susan, Liddy, and I assembled plants, books, lesson plans, and a few precious household items and departed for the West Coast. I would arrive in time to take a visiting professor job in Victoria, a short ferry boat ride away from Bellingham.

Leaving Mt. Pleasant was a heart-wrenching experience for some of us. Little Patti bore the brunt of our weepy disengagements. With Sue crowned the senior prom queen and her sister, Liddy, the queen's attendant, both girls had multiple friendships and activities. Katherine shared a house and deep attachments with five other girls in East Lansing, while my university colleagues felt like a second family to me.

Since Jim lived in a university apartment, barely large enough for two, finding a home in Portland was the next urgent step. We agreed to gather there as a family, with five children staying in Portland and Tim and Jim continuing their father-son duo as before. Mike's journal entry, which he shared with me, was prophetic, "there was no one there for me." Michael remained excluded from that inner circle.

Jim and I lived separated most of the week, deeply immersed in our work, so adapting to new living conditions posed less of a problem for me. But Mike and Patti were wholly unprepared for an urban school environment. Northeast Portland schools offered large, well-resourced programs with a sizable contingent of street-wise students, some of whom were active gang members—and not to be trifled with. Socially backward, Mike tried to stay clear of troublemakers but couldn't avoid the tough guys. Day after day, Mike was relieved of his lunch and cash in the boy's bathroom. While passive with peers, Mike acted out in the family, behaving erratically and refusing to obey or subdue his outbursts. Mike seemed constantly agitated, even on regular doses of Ritalin to help him with his ADHD.

Tim and his dad visited our Portland home regularly for that first year. While Jim and I reconnected with quiet talks, movies, and eating out, the two brothers were making mischief with the neighborhood girls across the street. I suppose this adolescent sex benefited the older brother, but Mike was over his head emotionally. Tim took advantage by preempting his younger brother's fumbling efforts with his masterful tactics. Mike would often come away disappointed and disjointed from the encounters.

Patti's turmoil continued with Mike in the home, and added to that, her stumbling efforts to succeed in that large grammar school of more than 900 students left her tormented. One day she came home sobbing; the second-grade teacher had taped her mouth shut because she was talking. I doubt Patti uttered a word that day the teacher punished her, given her ongoing trauma and inherent shyness. But it took a village to get that teacher fired, as the principal appeared disinterested in our story of abuse. Once I threatened to hire a lawyer and march into the courtroom with the parents of children the teacher had muffled with tape, the superintendent heard our plea.

My children's problems mounted; they needed help with their homework. Mike had been threatened on his way to school and needed a ride. Their orthodontist was on the other side of town and required hours of transport and waiting time. Shopping and dinner took more hours. How could I possibly earn tenure with these pressures?

At one point, Mike and Patti boarded the wrong bus and traveled for six hours throughout the city. Only after the bus pulled into its final stop did the driver notice the two frightened children cringing in the back seat. Undoubtedly, this episode started the rapid attrition of my bright idea that I could do it all: a new job and successful parenting.

After the bus incident, Mike vowed never to get lost again, taking a plunge into map making. He studied and created city maps of Portland,

Seattle, outlying towns, then turned to make Oregon maps of cities, mountains, and oceans. Then he discovered the stars of the stellar constellations, a spiritual experience. My son had finally stumbled into something that focused his brain and quieted his outbursts. He relished his geography classes, which quickly became his favorite subject.

Patti, however, was inconsolable those Portland years, deeply missing her older sister, and her dad, the linchpin of our family. Despite his chronic enabling of Mike, the children's father succeeded in controlling Mike's worst outbursts. Patti told me in an e-mail that her life during this time was unbearable.

"I distinctly remember one day crying uncontrollably while in elementary school in Portland. I missed Sue and Dad so much."

Did I even notice? How could such a state of affairs happen in our once orderly, loving family?

Troubled by the absence of Sue, who had eloped with her high school boyfriend, and her dad, living five hours away, Patti suffered deep depression, speaking little and being subject to tearful outbursts. I tried remedying the situation by taking in a foster girl, an older sister for Patti, a massive mistake. We were all in deep distress, but as the youngest, Patti took the biggest hit.

This new responsibility drained my energies further when I discovered that Diana was seriously out of control. Thirteen-year-old Diana brought older men into the house, flashed her body in Mike's presence, and stole money by forging checks, skillfully signing my name. I felt myself going under with the turmoil.

Reluctant to find still another foster home for this tormented girl, the social worker pressed me to try teaching her life skills; "she just needs more love," I recall her saying. After six months and worn out by her antics, Diana exited on the arm of her case manager. Her next stop was a group home for disturbed girls.

Portland looked like a dead end for my children. In addition, my father hoisted my younger schizophrenic sister, Sharon, into my care, thrusting my children into a whirlpool of insanity. Something had to change.

After two years, in desperation, I talked to Jim about moving the family to Bellingham, especially in light of the smaller schools. I sold my lovely 1927 built home, and we bought a larger house in Jim's bailiwick with a bus that stopped in front of the house to deliver the children wherever they might go. I planned to find a suitable apartment in Portland and do most of the commuting. I'd have plenty of time to get articles and perhaps even a book finished in time to earn tenure.

My income could help support the children for extracurriculars, as I no longer had family expenses. In agreeing to send a sizeable monthly payment for family maintenance, I needed to stay in low-cost housing and watch my pennies. I didn't realize how deprived I would feel since the situation looked ideal at the time. After years of feeling short-changed by living in rented rooms, I bought a small condo and purchased a beautiful townhome two years later.

CHAPTER NINETEEN

Parental Encounters

S haron's brilliant career lasted only six years before the downward spiral began. After being hospitalized, she returned to a lonely apartment without family connections in the area. I tried to warn my parents and wake them up from their emotional oblivion. I recalled occasions where they behaved less than rectitudinous, even beyond the pale.

I arrived in California fatigued at the end of a quarter, taking my spring break from teaching and parenting duties to be with them. After eating dinner in their upscale ranch house, I steeled myself, knowing a conversation about Sharon, alone in Chicago, would come up.

The great news—never spoken out loud—was that Mom's drinking had tapered off. She enjoyed retirement with Dad in California and found friends, activities, and church to be a happy round of accomplishments. The not-so-good news: Mom's health had become precarious, one infection after another, lots of fatigue and weakness.

"My swollen belly," she complained, "takes away my appetite. I don't know what's wrong, and the doctors can't figure out what's wrong with me either."

It was an odd turnaround: Dad's health was splendid, and he had never looked better, while Mom's energy kept dwindling. It didn't help that their last years living in Wilmette fostered even greater alcohol dependency and, later, illness for my mother. We had no idea she'd be gone in a few short years.

After Mom died at age 65, I discovered a long-forgotten photo of my parents. Retired in southern California, the couple appeared at ease with life and one another. Such a gratifying thought: my parents had reconciled after years of turmoil.

* * *

While my parents were still living in Wilmette and after I returned from Asia, I talked with Sharon, who confided that our parents were now involved in some drinking group, calling themselves "The Untouchables." "What could that mean?" I asked. Sharon believed the group had set themselves "above typical drinkers." We figured out this crowd took its name from an award-winning American crime drama on television that ran from 1959 to 1963. The program featured crime-fighting agents, headed by actor Robert Stack, who were handpicked for their courage, moral character, and incorruptibility.

These suburban untouchables applied the qualities of courage, morality, and virtue to their supposed capacity for drinking more in a single evening and "holding their liquor" more successfully than anyone they knew. What a travesty, I shuddered, especially in light of my mother's tendency for binge drinking that so quickly got out of control. And her drinking went on and on for decades. My mother's outrageous behavior was sometimes alarming, even dangerous. Still, I often suffered amnesia about her addiction, pretending everything was normal.

* * *

Encounters with my parents could be fraught with inappropriate, unkind, or even extreme outcomes.

Married in September, we decided to spend Christmas with my folks. Everyone appeared delighted to see the new couple and hear about our married life. I felt transformed, now viewing my childhood home as a refuge rather than a wrestling match.

A timid knock on my bedroom door. "What's up, I called from the bed."

"Just me," said my mother. I thought we could chat briefly now that the men are downstairs having breakfast."

"Sure, Mom."

I remember leaning on the closed door as Mom asked me question after question. "How are things going in your relationship with Jim?" I began to feel uncomfortable. Where was this going? I deflected her inquiries about our sex life with girlish giggling, which seemed enough of an answer. Then she popped out with:

"Your Dad hasn't touched me since you were married."

What could I say? What's more embarrassing than talking about your parents' love life? Shrugging it off, I offered her little consolation. I thought they both were too old, in their mid to late forties, to be sexually involved, anyway. The matter was dropped, and we never spoke of intimacies again.

As a young wife, unduly happy with married life and my three beautiful daughters, I pledged to visit my parents often, keeping the connection strong so the children could enjoy their grandparents. With my new life, again and again, I drew a curtain over my mother's alcoholism. I lived in a make-believe relationship with them, ignoring my mother's incapacity to relate and my father's ongoing rage and biting edge. I suspect he must have inflicted these on Sharon when he disapproved of her choices.

*　*　*

Our car pulled into the driveway of their new ranch-style home in Highland Park, a beautiful brick with my father's skilled landscaping enhancing the front yard. Our three small children, restless after the long drive, wanted out of the car: now. I swung out of the passenger seat to open up the back seat so they could clamber out, and I saw the look on my father's face: horror! Before I could get to the car handle, I heard him yell: "You're fat, my God, you've become fat!" I turned deliberately and, in a restrained tone, said, "No, Dad, you're wrong. I'm six months pregnant."

"My God, another pregnancy so close to these others. What's the matter with you?" Turning to my mother, I ignored that remark and began to chat about our long drive from Minnesota while Jim delivered the children from the car.

The rest of the visit focused on my mother's new interior decorating, a lackluster beige throughout the house: couch, chairs, carpets, and draperies. A minimalist kitchen discouraged me from offering to cook. As I recall, TV dinners were the standard cuisine. It made less fuss and muss in the kitchen.

* * *

On another occasion, my father's urgent voice told me I needed to come. "I've got important business, and Mom doesn't like to be alone in the house anymore. Here's the date and plane time."

'How about my kids, Dad?" "Bring them along. The kids will cheer her up."

I no sooner walked into my parents' house before I glimpsed Dad opening the closet to get his hat and coat, planning to leave abruptly. He appeared more tense than usual, barely said "hello" to me, and now he's gone. I walked to the front door to wave him off as he jumped into the taxi, but he didn't even give me a nod.

Preparing to relax after traveling with three children, I wasn't ready for the heavy sound of a door slamming. Now, what's with Mom? I understand she's mad at Dad, but she should at least come out and visit with the children.

Mom did not leave her bedroom that night or the next day. I was frantic, knocking, pleading with her to open the door. I didn't have Dad's phone number and wanted to avoid worrying Jim. What shall I do? I needed to compose myself. In the meantime, the children needed food and care and a quiet place to sleep.

On the third day, I knew something had to give. I smelled smoke oozing out of the bottom of her bedroom door and shaking from head to foot while banging on the door; I called the police—or maybe it was the fire department. I can only recall my terror when the officers broke the window, hauled my mother out of the room, while squashing out the burning cigarette in the mattress.

That's when I called my husband and asked for his advice. With Jim's trained investigative abilities, he located my father, gave him the bad news, and summoned him home.

*   *   *

Even sacred events resulted in catastrophe once my mother began drinking. "Who's on the phone, Jim," I called out. "Your Dad," he replied.

"Well, that's a shift. It's usually Mom who calls. I wonder what he wants."

"Hello, Dad, what's up? How are you doing?" Dad got right to the point. Your mother told me you couldn't afford to attend Dave's wedding. Your Mom is distraught because she bought dresses for the girls and wants them in Cincinnati for your brother's wedding. Dave finished his military stint in Korea, building and managing hospitals, recently received his Master's in Hospital Administration, and wants to gather the family to celebrate his marriage.

But I told you, Dad, we're strapped for funds. I can't ask my husband to take on any more debt. He's paying tuition now for me to complete my teaching degree. He's already exhausted from the additional job of teaching night classes at the Reformatory. That train ride from Minneapolis to Cincinnati is too costly for us."

OK, can you try this? You buy the train ticket and get the hotel room. After the wedding, I'll pay for that or any other expenses. You'll have a great time. And Mom will be thrilled to see the girls. And I know you want to see the happy couple, Dave and Ann." Jim nodded his OK, figuring out how to balance the monthly expenses.

The two families gathered in downtown Cincinnati for a festive evening at a local restaurant. My mother was ebullient with her arms around the two children—baby Liddy left at home as too young for the event—and Dad at his jovial self, greeting his son's bride, Ann, her parents, and older brother. We were seated at a round table when I noticed Mom behaving strangely. She looked irritated and feverish, probably with hot flashes, which flared up years after her surgery. Oh, oh, now she's fidgeting, "Mom, what's wrong?"

"I need to go to the ladies' room." She excused herself and disappeared. Because Ann's folks didn't drink, my Dad believed that a good host should pass up offering cocktails to the drinkers. A lull and my father pointed to me, "figure out what's happening with your Mom."

Mom, still in the restroom, seemed to be slurring her words. "Damn, I'm a mess. Just leave me alone. I'll be out in a minute."

Returning to the table, I used body language to Dad, signaling tummy upset, and we knew Mom was having trouble with her stress-related incontinence. So, back to the conversation. But still no Alice. Time for me to leave the table. I did find Mom—in the bar. When she saw me, she threw her latest martini down in one gulp and awkwardly gliding off the stool, she swerved toward me.

I assisted her into the booth, helped her negotiate the seating, and we returned to our conversation. Within 10 minutes, I saw Mom slide from her seat, slowly dragging her skirt behind her, and to my horror, fell under the table with her corset, garter belt, and legs exposed.

I knew the deal. Dad invited me to the wedding to ensure Mom wouldn't do any of this. And I failed him again. Dad was furious. I grabbed one of the oversized linen napkins, covered her exposed area, then plunged under the table to pull my mother out. Someone must have assisted me in getting her to the ladies' room, where I drenched her face with cold water, inadvertently soaking the front of her beautiful blue silk suit. Returning with my bedraggled mother and looking at the faces around the table, I could see the evening had ended for everyone.

"I want to talk to you, Nanette." Dad pulled me apart from the group the next day after the wedding and, nodding his head, indicated we were to have a conversation in his car. I smiled and sat in the passenger seat, expecting to receive the trip reimbursement he had promised.

Unexpectantly, he began shouting, "I'm not paying a penny for your trip up here, and you can damn well know that if you want to see us, you can pay your own way." I was shocked. I couldn't face Jim with this calamity. "But you have to;

you must. You absolutely have to. You said you would. I can't go home without money to pay Jim back for this trip," I sobbed.

I heard myself shriek. "I will not return home without the money." My father, probably fearful of attracting attention, reached into his pants pocket where he kept his roll of bills, pulled out some money, and threw it at me. Under his censorious gaze, I picked up bills and coins and departed from the car without speaking. My humiliation complete, the train trip home with my deflated little ones felt as though it had taken a hundred years.

I soldiered through this. But my father, angry for a fistful of reasons, consigned me—and undoubtedly my mother when they got home—to a measure of his humiliation.

That trip curtailed my interest in engaging with unloving parents, a resolve I soon forgot—until the next time they requested my presence.

After this egregious interaction with my father, I tried to recall when he was lighthearted, even somewhat funny. Viewing him in a positive light, even when he was severely distressed with me, gave me a measure of comfort. After all, I repeated to myself that he was my father, and I loved him. I fondly remember an interlude where he didn't play a trickster role or comment inappropriately. He was merely himself, a countryman at heart.

* * *

About a year after our return from Asia, my Dad decided to visit us, leaving my mother home with 16-year-old Dave. When Dad pulled up in a cab, I could see how jaunty he looked, jumping out of the car like a young man. How different from his usual glum appearance when he sees me.

"Hi, Dad," Jim called out. You're just in time to get in the car so we can make the show tonight. Dinner after at our favorite restaurant." During the drive into the city, Dad was all chatter about his sales meeting starting tomorrow, held at the Nation's Capital this year. As vice president of his company, he kept close tabs on all aspects of the business, especially sales.

"You'll love the program tonight, Dad. It's an international group from India featuring their native dances." I didn't tell him that the ticket cost set us back considerably. I guess we were trying to impress him. Dad sniffed, "You think I'll like that?" "Of course," I insisted.

The theater lobby was packed, but we pushed our way through the crowded lobby, located our choice balcony seats, and prepared for a long evening of entertainment. After spending a year in Japan attending the fascinating Kabuki performances, puppet shows, and other theatrical productions in Tokyo, I was prepped for all international programs.

The Indian dancers worked their sinewy magic, their hands and feet moving to the rhythm of the traditional music. A half-hour into the show, Dad spoke entirely too loudly! "Where in the world is this thing going?" "Shush, Dad," I whispered, mortified beyond expression. After another fifteen minutes, Dad was restless, twitching in his seat like a 10-year-old.

"What's the problem, Dad?"

"I can't take another minute of this. I'll wait in the lobby for you."

Intermission. We poured out of the theater and found Dad standing at the door. "Are you two going to continue with another hour of this stuff?"

Jim and I exchanged looks. He's our guest. I guess we'd better call it a wrong choice and move on.

"I'm sorry, Dad," I said smugly. I thought you'd enjoy the experience of high culture."

"Oh, that's what it is. No wonder I don't like it!"

How could my Dad sour my entire evening with his pedestrian tastes?

Driving home to Bethesda with Dad in the back seat, Jim looked at Dad in the rear-view mirror and commented. "You saved my bacon this evening. I could barely stand that program another minute either." The two men laughed heartily. My ego punctured, I retorted: "too bad you low-life types don't appreciate the higher culture." More male laughter was their only response.

* * *

At the dinner table with my parents, I squirmed because I knew what was coming: this dreaded conversation about Sharon's situation, whatever it was, and figuring out what to do about it. Maybe nobody knew what to do.

"Mom and Dad, listen to me," I said. "I'm telling you. Sharon's behavior is strange, abnormal. Dad, you were with her at the University Hospital when she had that first psychotic breakdown at 27. It's five years since then, and we know she must be alone and scared in Chicago. She doesn't answer the phone. She avoids seeing us when we visit and even runs away when she knows we're there. That's happened three times; the same thing happened to Dave. She sometimes forgets what she's saying. She seems lost and frightened. The last time we got together, she yelled at the children. I'm not sure she's eating regularly."

My parents glowered at me as though I was the crazy one. They felt confident that the early intervention was a one-time experience; after that psychiatric intervention, Sharon returned safely to her normal state. This was in the early years of relocating hospitalized mental patients from institutional care into local communities where most were unlikely ever to see a mental health professional. Mental health experts assured my parents that Sharon was cured.

I said differently. "She's getting progressively worse and may be doing even more poorly since you left the Chicago area and now lacks family or friends to support her. I know you helped her with that first intervention, but it didn't seem to work. Can't anything be done to support her?"

My last words faded as Dad jumped up from the table, knocking his chair to the floor.

"You don't know what you're talking about!" he said, launching into a tirade. "You're the troublemaker around here, not Sharon! She's being taken care of just fine, thank you," he shouted. "I send her all the money she needs."

"What! Is it my fault?" my Irish Catholic mother, guilty by birth, stammered. "Are you accusing me? Everything always seems to be my fault."

"That will be enough talk about Sharon. Case closed," Dad shouted.

Nothing changed, including their inability to maintain boundaries with my family and me.

CHAPTER TWENTY

Welcome to Bedlam

Sharon!

Storming through our Portland, Oregon, home day and night, I knew my sister must leave. Her insanity cut like a knife through our lives. Finally, I faced the phone call I'd been dreading. After our agreement, Dad needed to keep his word for me to bring Sharon from Chicago to my home, where he would take care of the rest: fly up from California and take my sister home with him. I left that message on his phone a week ago, and he still hasn't returned the call. Why was he stalling? Sharon was ready to go. I was ready to shove her out.

We had made a deal. Dad proposed: "You told your Mom last Sunday, when you called, that you plan to be at your sociology conference in Chicago. Why not bring Sharon back with you after you finish? You're the one who mentioned she's too alone there in the big city. Once she's on the West Coast, I'll fly up from San Diego. It's only a short hop away. You can do this for me. I'm too old now for that long flight to Chicago, and Anne can't travel that far either. She gets too nauseated from flying."

"Ok, Dad, I'll let you know when I have Sharon safely in my home," I agreed as his reassuring words murmured in my ears.

Now, I'm trying to follow up on his promise to pick up my poor, deranged sister. After about five minutes of an inane phone conversation, he finally blurted out: "I can't take your sister. Anne can't be expected to care for Sharon in her elderly years. She's been very involved with her beloved granddaughter, who's over here half the time. Sharon will be fine with you and your family. You know, I'm not married to her mother."

"What are you saying, Dad? I've barely moved to Portland, and you lay this assignment at my door. I'm making every effort to establish myself and the kids: new city, demanding job, difficult colleagues, and Jim five hours away in Bellingham. We have a commuting marriage now. Taking on Sharon would make this an untenable situation."

Perhaps I had an ill-conceived vision, but I had dreamed of Sharon, intact and happy, living in sunny California, keeping up her beautiful tan, and meeting eligible men. Anne was part of the fantasy. That gracious lady, an absolute jewel, would look after my precious sister and bring her back to health. We could all visit together once Sharon returned to normality.

I made more phone calls with the same message. "You have to take Sharon. Keeping her here is unthinkable."

But Dad was not budging. "You know, I'm not married to her mother." And then a final closure. "Don't call me anymore about this. You heard me. I cannot take Sharon. My answer is no!"

What a lame excuse... "not married to her mother." I could not believe he kept repeating that ridiculous phrase to me. My mind raced with the injustice of it all.

First, my father tried to unload my mother on me, and now he's doing the same thing with my sister. I vowed last year, during our family turmoil, that my only wish was to keep my family calm and happy once our lives slowed down. How could I possibly achieve that by looking after Sharon?

I brought her back, shocked and disgusted by my father's deceit. I couldn't manage her. He deserted us both and abandoned Sharon, the same stunt he pulled when he left Chicago and retired in California. Our parents left her behind. What kind of parents do that? He expected me to understand him, but he had no idea what I was going through. He left me holding the bag, a bag I was terrified to look inside.

And he used his second wife as the reason he couldn't take care of Sharon. Why me? I knew nothing about the adult Sharon or how to help her. My nerves were in shreds realizing that my father made the situation normal for himself while he *threw* me to the wolves.

* * *

After arriving in Chicago for the conference, I encountered a series of mishaps and disasters. Once the plane landed, I rushed to my hotel, took a quick shower, registered for the sociology conference and evening festivities, and located Sharon's apartment on the near North Side. I planned to visit her the following day when we were both fresh and rested.

On a bitterly cold December morning, I hastily grabbed a cab to Sharon's apartment, some considerable dollars away from my hotel, and knocked on her dingy apartment door, jumping from one foot to another to warm up. No answer. I took a quick taxi back and read my carefully crafted research paper to a yawning audience. Feeling defeated, I rushed again to her apartment. Silence. The door remained shut tight against me.

Time seeped away. I felt anguished that I had taken on this clearly impossible job while trying to set up a new home, build my career, and seek tenure in an urban university. The kids needed me to help them put down roots in their new schools and neighborhood and to support the teenagers in their search for part-time jobs. The biggest hurdle turned out to be negotiating family time together on weekends. Jim and I faced the looming prospect of bringing the two parts of our fragmented family together on infrequent weekends and holidays.

It did seem crazy to take this long-distance position in Portland. Jim and I took turns commuting from his base in Bellingham, Washington, but his free time was minimal as an administrator. In the beginning, Jim did the commuting because traveling with the children complicated our situation. After I moved the children to Bellingham and got an apartment, it was my turn to commute. At least once or twice a month, I took the five-hour drive after working all week, easing onto the road around 9 p.m. on a Friday for our bi-weekly visits. Because of the prohibition on nepotism, the lack of a teaching position in my area, and Jim's inability to take time away from his job, I took on most of the commuting. An unspoken taboo in academic circles involved hiring a married couple.

So, what choice did I have to salvage my hard-won Ph.D. and prove myself? Live in Bellingham, unemployed? Or take my first choice: the opportunity to use my training and skills? At age 44, a very late start, I took on a new academic position as an associate professor of sociology. I had no time to spare in building a career. With the children settled in their various schools, I was ready to take on the world!

* * *

Once again, I faced Sharon's bleak door, brushing snow off my coat onto the filthy hall rug. It was the third and final day of trying to reach her, or I would fly home without getting her to open the door.

"I can't do this, Sharon!" I screamed. "Open the goddamn door, or I'll call the police!"

Again, total silence. Fearing the worst—seeking police action—I tearfully ran down the three floors and begged the landlord to open Sharon's door. He explained it was against company policy but seemed eager to comply if only I took her out of there. Quick.

Sharon had five deadlocks, each more stubborn than the one before. He grunted harshly with late-stage emphysema as he climbed the three flights of stairs. Bent over, gasping, he began the process of opening the door.

Once in the room, I took in the horror of Sharon's illness. My sister sat on a torn sofa staring at a cloudy television, her back supported by a threadbare pillow, dirty socks on her smelly feet. Her hair hadn't been washed in days, maybe weeks. She wore a food-spattered t-shirt with the heat turned up to 85 degrees.

This can't be Sharon. It must not be Sharon. My God, how could this happen? How *did* this happen?

I took another look around. I saw papers strewn around the small studio, but one large pile caught my attention: uncashed checks sent from our generous but deceptive father, who hoped to smooth matters over by sending money once he moved West. He never knew what happened to those checks.

"Hi, Nanette," Sharon hoarsely greeted me. "You look great. I love your jacket. You always look so good. And you have a new hairstyle."

Before I could respond, Sharon lapsed into a catatonic state, resuming her fixed position in front of the soundless and blank television. As I suspected, the kitchen was bereft of anything resembling food if I didn't count the gummy candies stuck to the countertop.

I found myself sweating in Chicago's sub-zero weather. My head throbbed with the same heaviness I'd had for days. I couldn't call Dad because he was unsympathetic. Jim was dutifully involved with his new dean's job, and anyway, he thought this undertaking a mission impossible. I had to find a solution on my own.

OK, so much for the sociology conference, I thought to myself. I can't make any points with this situation hanging over my head. Let's feed the girl and figure out how to move her to the airport.

I laid out my strategy carefully, knowing Sharon would be positive about seeing my growing family "just for a few days, of course."

"Let's have dinner first," I said cheerily. "Then we can talk about you visiting the kids. I saw a restaurant on my way here. How do steak and fries sound?"

Each step to getting Sharon off the couch and to the restaurant was arduous. Finding clean clothes for Sharon in her filthy apartment. Sliding on the icy sidewalks to the eatery. Ordering the food. Eating the food. All were exhausting steps for Sharon, and she balked at each move.

"I'm too tired, Nanette. I can't eat now; I'm not hungry."

I, on the other hand, was determined.

"OK, Sharon, I know, but I'm starved, and I need to share a meal with you after all these years. Remember how Dad used to cook the beef to perfection?"

The food was ordinary, the company grim, the eating spasmodic. I gave up after a few bites and asked for doggie bags.

Over the next two days, I enticed Sharon into different diners down the street. Back at her place, we sorted out clothes, called for an extra air ticket from Chicago to Portland, and packed her out of that appallingly grimy apartment she called "home." I thought all was well when we finally arrived at the airport.

But not for long.

"I need to go to the bathroom, Nanette. I'll be right back."

What was I thinking? I let her go alone in the vast Chicago airport. Ten minutes, 15, 20, and 25 minutes passed without a sign of her. An hour later, I was steaming, running from one ladies' room to another and finding no sign of her.

Sharon was gone.

Why not try the United Airlines desk? I thought. The airline broadcasts names, and she could find me at our gate.

I let a gate clerk know my predicament and plopped down on the seat closest to the gate.

"Sharon Trexler," I soon heard. "Please meet your party at the United Desk, Gate 15."

It's only a matter of time now, I thought.

But with the clock ticking frantically, I realized Sharon could be seriously lost. Given her severe hallucinations, I pictured her crouched in a corner, terrified—and our plane was due to board in half an hour.

Next plan: contact the airport police for a missing, mentally ill woman, and give them the following description.

"Dark-haired, 39-year-old woman wearing a black coat, black boots, and red-orange ski cap," I told the officer. "She's been missing for nearly two hours in the Chicago O'Hare Airport and answers to the name, 'Sharon.' She is friendly but very confused."

Twenty minutes later, two beefy policemen escorted Sharon to the gate and, taking no chances, accompanied us into the waiting airplane. The beloved police officers stood at our seats until Sharon strapped herself into the seat. I relaxed at last.

Barely an hour into the flight, Sharon poked my arm.

"I have to go to the bathroom. My period's starting."

This time I am on to her ditch-and-disappear game. Vowing to keep matters under control, I insisted on going with her, only to realize, when she stood up, that the back of her trousers was slick with blood. Our luggage was out-of-reach in cargo.

Frantically, I pulled out my make-up kit, books, papers, and pens from my overstuffed carry-on bag and located the extra pair of panties I invariably stow away when I travel. Force marching my charge ahead of me down the too-long aisle, we encountered puzzled looks from passengers as I gripped tightly to her waist.

Once we located the toilet and slipped inside, I briskly washed the blood off Sharon's body and clothes. Finally, I squeezed overtight underwear and wet pants onto her stiff, resistant body. I felt some inkling of what lay in store for me once I arrived home.

CHAPTER TWENTY-ONE

No Solutions for Sharon

O ne morning soon after we arrived in Portland, my children reported the bad news about living with our new visitor.

"Mom, I can't sleep a wink with Sharon's prowling and shrieking all night. She hogs up the bathroom, and I need a shower before going to work," eighteen-year-old Liddy complained.

"Me, too, and I'm scared of Auntie Sharon," echoed seven-year-old Patti.

What could I do? Even with cramming five children into an admittedly spacious three-bedroom house, built in 1927 to last, and then putting 13-year-old, unpredictable, moody Mike in a makeshift room in the basement next to the ancient furnace, I still did not have a private space for Sharon.

I felt especially concerned about Mike, who was so dependent on his father and brother. Tim had moved with his dad to Bellingham, leaving Mike behind with me. Both boys had been well-supported at the public schools we left behind, but missing both his brother and Dad, Mike seemed riddled with anxiety in this new urban school.

When we lived in Mt. Pleasant, Jim used to take him out daily for "prizes" to quell his outbursts. With Daddy no longer with him daily, Mike suffered deprivation, and I couldn't appease him.

"My Dad always spoils me," Mike would write years later, "and I get my way, usually against my mother's will. I always want to go to the store and get a prize or something. I think he knows I have great sensitivity and mood swings as a kid. Always laughing and crying in a short period of time. Always the imbalances in the same moment."

But what could I do about 13-year-old Mike when Sharon's outbursts took center stage? And Sharon roamed—especially at night. She went up and down the creaky stairs, howling and screaming obscenities repeating her baby-talk litany.

"Hersee, Himsee, Hersee, Himsee," her voice became more desperate with each utterance.

Breakfast wasn't much better. On a bitterly cold February day, I served her scrambled eggs and toast to warm up what she complained was her "cold tummy." Mike crashed into the kitchen nook, upsetting Sharon's coffee and fragile equilibrium. The eggs went soft and weepy as Sharon resumed the previous night's irrational rant.

"Sharon, you need some medication to help you sleep and keep you from being so agitated," I gently told her.

Rage followed rage, as foot-stamping and shouting, Sharon bolted from any room when I tried to raise the medication issue.

But I had other roles to play, and Sharon occupied only part of my existence. My new position required my best energy. University classes at Portland State were both large and demanding. Still, I was in glory land with my adult students, many of whom had their own fascinating histories.

After living in small towns in Minnesota and Michigan, I embraced the vibrant city of Portland. It was almost like being in love: the trees, theaters, restaurants, fountains, good film center, and above all, the people. When I first arrived, I often laughed out loud with joy. I felt elated by the warm, friendly, easygoing urban center with personality and heart.

After Sharon moved in, I found myself wrung out at the end of each day with the absurd regimen I had unwittingly taken on and lingered on Robert Frost's words: "and miles to go before I sleep." It became increasingly apparent Mike needed closer supervision than my schedule allowed, but it was months before Jim and I realized that Mike's stability had been badly compromised.

Too much had happened all at once: the family separation, my inability to hold things together on the home front, Sharon's disruptive influence, and the new school situation. We decided to move Mike to his Dad's apartment in Bellingham, where he began to thrive again with a smaller high school and his brother Tim's help supervising the rattled boy.

In those early days of our Portland life, everyone seemed to be in turmoil. The shift from our Michigan home took its toll. I made every effort to normalize our new life, but I was harried and overworked. Still, we set aside time for the children and me to be together.

Take a typical dinner, for instance, hardly a relaxing event, although enjoyed with relish by all. Undoubtedly, the children ate every morsel of food left in the fridge, so I would pick up the basics after work: chicken, potatoes, veggies, salad, and dessert. We needed more milk for breakfast, and I must not forget the healthy cereal and bread. I checked off my list.

Once home, I gathered the dirty laundry and ran two loads while cooking the new potatoes and chilling the mixed salad. On one particular night, I recall we ate broiled chicken, everyone's favorite, and squeaky green beans; only I enjoyed beans *al dente*. Conversation flowed. Everyone reported on their day.

Our evening was a happy one since the holiday vacation would begin soon, and there were plans to have Dad and Tim join us and lend a joyous spirit to the upcoming Christmas celebration. Next came dishes, then lecture writing, and bed at 2:00 a.m. The following day, I was up at 8:00 a.m. to get Patti and Mike fed and off to the nearby grammar school of nearly 900 students. Jim and I loved the fact many students were African American, an ethnic diversity so different from the small, all-white communities the children had experienced before.

Uncle Verdan, my father's brother, was one bright spot that softened the tension of Sharon's abrupt transfer into my life. I met my Uncle Verdan shortly after we moved into our Portland home in 1975. He called one Saturday and offered to come over and check out any needed repairs for the house. The house required outdoor painting, the gutters needed cleaning, maybe replacement, the plumbing showed signs of wear, and the windows needed a good wash. "Just up my alley," he said with a smile. I was delighted.

I wondered what family he had grown up in. Not a snide remark in sight. The children loved him and sat on the outdoor lawn as their great-uncle painted the entire house methodically, from top to bottom, that summer of 1976. I almost felt guilty, but he insisted on doing it for free. I compensated in a small way with food and other goodies he found heartwarming. That's how I came to describe our sweet uncle: heartwarming. He must have been in his eighties.

The first sign of my uncle's changed condition came from my father. Sometime that autumn or winter, his wife collapsed in the night on her way to the bathroom. When that dear lady died, Verdan died with her. He no longer called and refused to answer his phone. I had no way of reaching him.

Along with my siblings, Dad's words and conduct carried weight; in fact, he exerted considerable influence throughout all our lives. My father even confided in me at a low point in his life after his brother died suddenly. It appears contradictory that he and I should have a cordial relationship after all my father's manipulations and unrealistic expectations.

"Verdan died last night. I just heard from his daughter that the funeral would be held there in Portland. Could I stay with you in your apartment?"

We sat in my cozy kitchen at the rented table I turned in after the end of the school year, saving on rent while spending delicious summers at home. Our conversation had a surreal quality as Dad talked. Shaken by the loss of my uncle, I understood this event had triggered Dad's concern and his wish to have emotional support, spending more time with me instead of planning the typical hotel stay when traveling out of town.

"I can't believe my brother would let himself die, just die, because his wife had a stroke. She always had health problems. He was strong as a horse. He didn't have to die. He could have come to California and spent time with me. I insisted on this after her funeral, but he rejected my offer. He just said, 'I'm next, Van. I'm too lonely to go anywhere or do anything. My life just went downhill after her death. Thanks anyway.'"

Despite my sadness, I attempted to console Dad, but he seemed unable to accept his loss or grief. He continued with this sorrowful litany the entire time we spent together, except when he attended a large gathering of Verdan's relatives and friends, who thought I was my father's "date." Not a good joke, really, under the circumstances.

*   *   *

Extricating Sharon from our home was no easy task. The children pushed me to "do something about Sharon." What could I do? She refused to budge out of the house; she avoided open doors; she disappeared into the bathroom when she saw me preparing to leave the house. I was open to any plan to get her help and restore peace in the household.

One day, following my 2:00 p.m. lecture in criminology, an Amazonian-proportioned woman approached me with an oversized hand in greeting.

"Hi, I'm Kathleen," she announced, "and I work full time in the Benton County police force. It's hard to make every class if I'm on duty, so what can I do to pass the course?"

I assured her I could cover the missed material in an office hour that fit her schedule. We instantly bonded. After a few more conversations, I impulsively hugged Kathleen as my friend for life. I realized she could help me extract Sharon from my home and end the chaos she created.

The plan was flawless. Kathleen pulled together five friends, two of whom were also sister police officers. The children, safely installed in school, would not witness what appeared to be an act of betrayal. Our charming older home had multiple doors leading to gardens and walks. Kathleen assigned a person to guard each entry, so Sharon could not bolt. She wisely contacted a mental health officer she knew from her department. I had the Judas task of pointing out the culprit and embracing her in front of the many witnesses.

I called Sharon from the large airy bedroom she shared with Liddy and Patti. Without protest, she came downstairs—it was one of Sharon's rare, peace-loving days. The doorbell rang, and six women trooped in to nab the offender and "talk sense" so she would go peacefully to the mental health center and start her antipsychotic medications. But having descended to the front hall, she was startled as the doorbell rang again, and a husky male police officer entered. After one hard look at the mass of strangers, especially the gun-carrying officer, Sharon began her strange, otherworldly screech.

"Hersee, Himsee, Hersee, Himsee!"

I reached out, hoping to calm her down, but inadvertently became the victim as Sharon jumped on my back with considerable force and knocked me to the floor.

That did it. The gentle but irretrievably mad wrongdoer, handcuffed into surrender and suddenly transformed into a criminal, was hauled off to a locked mental health cell. The police report erroneously stated: "Violent female attacks sister, possession of weapon (gun), and had to be subdued."

Sharon never possessed a gun, of course, on that critical day of her banishment, but without "possession of weapon," it would have been more difficult to force her into care, given the state mental health laws. The special-trained police officer who rescued us knew precisely what kind of criminal charge would stick, allowing the patient to receive treatment.

Over the years, Sharon both flourished and languished, eventually disappearing from the mental health system I had so profoundly counted on to provide her stable support. As that system failed, my caregiving burdens increased.

CHAPTER TWENTY-TWO

A Perilous Path

Sharon did not settle into a healthy, regular routine. Instead, even with extensive mental health intervention, she had a series of "accidents." Were these accidents self-imposed or the outcome of her inability to control her life? It seemed she had one continuous disaster: breaking a left leg, badly scabbing both knees, injuring her right foot, and bruising her face. One day she showed up with a bad limp. I dreaded what could come next. I felt helpless to prevent her accidents. Why did I feel so responsible for whatever happened to her? I heard my father's voice.

"You're the one in charge. Now! Take care of it!"

But Sharon had her inner directives: demonic voices that provoked visions of profound horror.

Disaster soon arrived, including two suicide attempts—twice jumping off the Burnside Bridge that spans the Willamette River in Northwest Portland. Sharon leaped over the railing on the first attempt, smashed into the water, surfaced next to a startled family leisurely paddling their new rowboat, and was miraculously rescued almost immediately, without injury. Sharon appeared none the worse physically from her perverted adventure, shrugging off my concerns about her negative moods. Although growing up two short blocks from Lake Michigan, Sharon never learned to swim a stroke.

"Get off my back, Nanette. I'm just fine. You're a nag, do you know that? Just let me be."

But Sharon's depression seemed to be deepening. I decided to spend more time with her, trying to gauge her moods, inviting her to our home for daily dinners or frequent evenings out to movies or local events. Meanwhile, my children missed the intimacy of their mom around the kitchen table. We shifted to "formal" dinners with Sharon in our beautiful blue draperied dining room, hoping to fully embrace her as family. The intensive caregiving came to naught. Sharon continued down her singular path.

Three months later, the second jump at nearly the exact same bridge location broke her back but not her spirit. She suffered multiple fractures, and with her back confined in a brace, Sharon underwent a remarkable transformation: the mental symptoms disappeared. How could she survive that leap with such severe injuries?

Her niece, Kathy, generously gave Sharon her new-to-you bright orange coat acquired at the local Senior Center the afternoon before. This ancient wrap had an exquisite silk lining that, aside from warmth, had buoyancy that somehow held Sharon up long enough for the Coast Guard rescue boat to pick her up on that fateful Monday.

The hospital phone call stunned me into action. Outraged and gritting my teeth, I dashed over to the hospital, hastily leaving my students without notice, and once escorted into Sharon's room, began spewing out five reasons why Sharon should NEVER, NEVER, NEVER try that stunt again: *you're playing God; it's against the law; you've got many years ahead of you; I am devastated by worry and grief about these suicide attempts; the children have accepted you as part of our family.* Nodding her head vigorously from her intensive-care hospital bed, Sharon promised to wait for the "hand of God" to let her know when her time was up.

Once released and under the doctor's orders, she resumed a "normal" working schedule to strengthen her back. Up at 7:30, breakfast at the local diner, and then walking a specified route from 8:30 until noon, when she stopped for lunch at a different restaurant every day. At 1:00 sharp, the walking continued up and down the hills and parks of Portland until 5:00 p.m. Returning to her lovely upscale Northwest apartment I had located and furnished, Sharon acted happy and content with her back brace firmly in place. I seriously doubt the doctor had such a strenuous regime in mind when emphasizing that his patient should "take daily walks."

The post-suicide period was Sharon's happiest stretch. Unbelievably, for a brief moment, a completely sane Sharon emerged—a fascinating, well-educated, humorous woman—a delight to be with on any occasion: a film, family party, or an evening of "girl talk." How I relished getting to know this intelligent, multi-faceted sister of mine.

One of our favorite pursuits in which we both took delight was our Thursday night movie, usually at one of Portland's excellent neighborhood theaters. Sharon loved comedy: identified with the comic, mimicked the comic, and became entangled in the funny situation.

So, off we went to the Bagdad Theater in SE Portland one early spring evening to see "The Gold Rush," one of Charlie Chaplin's more side-splitting, ever-absurd films. My enjoyment bubbled up with joy over Sharon's ability to be in the moment, embracing the fun and nonsense of it all. Sharon was beside herself, rollicking with laughter as Chaplin poured salt on his boot, devoured the only food available in the frigid North, and tidied up his cabin with his splay-footed swagger.

A year after I brought Sharon to Portland, our father decided it might be time to step in and provide assistance now that Sharon had been integrated into the Oregon mental health system and appeared safe from harm. Cranky from travel and unaccustomed care responsibilities, Dad and his sweet-natured Anne arrived in Portland to serve as resident babysitters. They agreed to look after Mike and Patti, allowing me to travel with daughter Liddy for a weeklong criminology conference and two weeks playing tourist in Europe.

This time I attended every session in London, took copious notes, and did the academic dance of meeting and greeting colleagues. Liddy and I continued our journey across Europe, cavorting to Vienna, Rome, and Amsterdam. Invited to stay with a charming Dutch family, Liddy quickly found a job and a boyfriend, living in the Netherlands for two years.

* * *

Brace removal day. A few days after her back was completely healed, Sharon shifted abruptly. The hallucinations—voices screaming nonstop threats—could not be quieted, even with antipsychotic medication and talk therapy. Sharon was bereft of reason and quickly lost her way, whether walking through once-familiar neighborhoods in Portland or visiting us in Bellingham on winter or summer vacations.

I suffered a second round of emotional blows, when I perceived Sharon's catastrophic spiral becoming the new normal. I remember well this transformation as Sharon came tumbling down from her sanity perch to the depths below.

We knew we had lost her presence at our frequent family celebrations the Christmas she left her suitcase—with all her medications—on the train. Within two days, Sharon's disconnect vacillated between rage and withdrawal. The mental health system in Oregon proved futile—this was a holiday weekend—and despite multiple calls, I could not reach her therapist or contact Amtrak to locate her bag in time. The suitcase arrived a week later, the same day as her departure back to Portland.

Here's a scene from that Bellingham holiday dinner in 1978 that featured Sharon without her medication. The call to dinner—where is Sharon? I'd better send Mike, our handsome son. He loves any special attention.

"Mike, you run downstairs and get Sharon for our holiday dinner. She loves turkey with cranberries and mashed potatoes."

Sixteen-year-old Mike returned, but without Sharon.

"She can't come now." "Why not?" I insist. "She doesn't have anything to wear," Mike responded.

We all had in mind she lacked a festive outfit. So, I yelled downstairs where the larger nest of bedrooms in our expansive split-level home was located:

"Sharon, you're OK, come and join us."

A few minutes later, wild-eyed, hair snarled and matted, a faint stench suggestive of used clothing and ragged pajamas, an un-showered Sharon emerged from her hideout. "Hi, everyone," she called out. The table of 25 adults and children stared, appalled, then looked away until I hesitantly reached out and hugged her, and the tension dissolved. Everyone relaxed and cried out, "Hi, Sharon," and the dinner was off to a fine start.

I can't say I was cheerful about Sharon's disorganized state—appearances can be deceiving. But finally, after a slow acceptance, I had to admit that regardless of how I felt, neither I nor anyone else had control over my sister's behavior. Once I put her on the return train to Portland that holiday, I felt only overpowering relief that Sharon was on her own, leaving me to relax and enjoy the rest of the family vacation, unencumbered by Sharon's disturbing actions.

The drama continued but took different turns over the years, especially Sharon's regular "runs" from public housing for a variety of reasons—fear of the manager, new management, different social worker assigned to her case, a cold room, a hot room, drunks in the hallway, and on and on. After chasing her around the neighborhood, sometimes, too often for my well-being, another family member or I found her behind or even inside a garbage can connected with restaurants she habitually visits. Undoubtedly, my sister sought a shelter that would hold her snugly against her fears.

One of Sharon's garbage-can episodes remains etched in our family memory. After nearly three weeks of being missing, Sharon had moved into the category of "homeless," the police choosing not to pursue the more insistent classification of "missing person," which provided resources for official searches.

After the massive release of mental patients from institutions a few decades back, society abandoned the idea of caring for the mentally deranged. Instead, they were "free"—free to wander, free to be victims, free to be "public nuisances," or even free to die on city streets.

It remained up to our family to carry out the intrepid task of finding Sharon before she succumbed to what we concluded would only be a heartrending end.

"Sharon, where are you? Tim shouted as he scoured Portland's northwest neighborhoods on his bike.

"She can't have gone far," insisted Jim, who combed the streets by car looking for a trace of the missing woman with little Patti's help.

"Sharon, damn it, why are you doing this? You'll be kicked out of your apartment for sure now and have no place to go," I muttered aloud to no one.

Suddenly, mid-afternoon of the fourth day of our grueling search, a gleeful laugh as Tim bellowed out:

"I found Sharon over here behind the Rose Restaurant. She was hiding in their dumpster, but her coat got stuck, so I had to help pull her out. Sorry, she's got some gunk on her clothes I couldn't brush off."

Once we gathered, I wanted to give prodigal Sharon a tongue-lashing: I'm-so-frigging-mad-at-you-lecture. But we were entirely too happy to do anything but hug her.

Unpredictable and frequent departures from her public housing meant Sharon lost whatever tenuous link she had to earthly security: a place to live, friends, furniture, television, and even priceless keepsakes. This necessitated my locating another, usually even more squalid dwelling, newly equipped with a bed, dresser set, television, wall pictures, and kitchen wares. Starting over each time, I realized landlords' reluctance to rent to the mentally ill, as Sharon was now a security liability.

On a scorching hot day in Portland in late May, I am sitting on a non-air-conditioned bus, again scouring the town for low-income housing available for the mentally ill. Taking a bus around Portland in this heat seemed easier than driving and looking for an elusive parking place. Sure enough, Sharon's last run left her, once again, with a two-week eviction notice. So little time to pull off another housing miracle.

It had to be the right location—Sharon insisted on only two urban areas she was willing to live in—Northwest or Downtown Portland. You must not forget the right price—it needed to stay within the Social Security disability funding limits. And don't overlook the right balance of residents. The public housing office required a diversity of renters: a mix of genders, ages, and levels of disability, rather than a concentration of the mentally ill. I could not seek private housing because these units typically lacked mental health supervision. "It's a bummer," my daughter Katherine would say about these housing searches.

The bus pulled over, my hand gripping the burning hot support pole. This was my fifth stop. This time I'm also exploring outlying areas, such as Southeast Portland. I noticed that gentrification was beginning slowly in this neighborhood, but most of the available apartments still looked unbelievably small and dingy, with windows not washed in years. Sharon will have to be adaptive, or we're left with the mental health system warehousing her in what could be an unacceptable apartment. The problem there: she would have no mental health watchdog. I returned home defeated.

The call came the following day. An apartment meeting the required housing specifications would be available in four days. I wondered what had happened to the last resident. I quickly moved forward, notifying the mental health center so Sharon could claim it. Not a bad spot: downtown Portland, fourth floor, elevator, a studio with a few windows, a small kitchen, right in the immediate downtown, six easy blocks to Sharon's mental health building, and about four blocks from my office.

I rounded up another bed, dresser, television, and kitchen items. Thank heavens for the St. Vincent de Paul charitable organization! We were all set once Sharon approved. My burden was lifted. I spent the following weekend happily with my family in Bellingham, going through the rounds of faculty parties.

The roller-coaster ride with Sharon continued from 1975, when I first rescued her from her dilapidated Chicago apartment, through 1991, when I escaped to Australia with my Fulbright Scholar Award secured tightly in my briefcase. Early retirement from Portland State University with bonuses and settling in Bellingham with my family after 16 years of commuting and limited visiting had been my wish for years.

The 1992 Fulbright travel grant and sabbatical salary for half a year allowed for research work in Australia over the next three winters, ensuring I had genuinely lost Sharon. Over the months I was absent from Portland, she neither wrote nor called to make contact. Once I was home, I kept up occasional visits after returning from Australia to ensure Sharon was comfortable. Not until I had a crisis in Bellingham did I stop the visits.

On August 1, 1998, Jim woke to a hot, sunny day clutching his chest and breathing hard, the classic symptoms of a heart attack. More severe heart attacks and strokes followed, ending his brilliant lecturing and writing career. I entered four years of intensive caregiving and full-time teaching to hold our life together. Exhausted by my job and caregiving, I could no longer reach out to Sharon.

*   *   *

Fast forward to 2006. Through sister Marilyn's deep search and strong urgings, I found Sharon now constrained in a notorious "One Flew Over the Cuckoo's Nest" setting. Unable to be released until a guardian and appropriate housing could be found, the authorities now recognized Sharon required close supervision. My new role as legal guardian began.

In a surprise shift, Sharon had retreated differently than the more familiar runs. Instead of scurrying through alleys to ease her fears, she took an opposite tack to cope with life. She shut herself up for years in one of those paint-scarred, broken-windowed hotel rooms where the destitute cluster: the very poor, more deeply disabled, and abandoned mentally ill patients.

Lacking a bathtub or shower in her rundown hotel, Sharon could not keep herself clean. She became a target for lice, bedbugs, and other repulsive creatures that feed on hapless humans. The smell must have alerted the authorities because, after months of Sharon's social isolation, the hotel manager summoned the police. Sharon soon found herself inside the least accessible confinement facility, effectively cutting out family support.

CHAPTER TWENTY-THREE

Buried Evidence

How could I be expected to know or understand what Sharon had gone through with her mental illness? After all, she reappeared in my life in 1975, at thirty-nine-years old. What can you know about a person, with only occasional visits and great distances between us? The bigger question: why did I step in at this late date and become her keeper?

I was not the first family member attempting to rescue Sharon. Our sister, Marilyn, now married and living in Canada, unwittingly stepped into the savior role. In 1962, Marilyn had just had a new baby, and with three more children, six years and under, I know she must have felt swamped. Full steam ahead, and with little notice and less baggage, Sharon arrived at Marilyn's place in the midst of the turmoil, having decided to make the dramatic decision to stay with their family until she could "get settled" into a new life.

Exhausted from new baby demands and lack of sleep, Marilyn brought our beleaguered sister into her home for over two months, eventually finding her a nearby apartment, a congenial roommate, and a job. For weeks Marilyn worked with "incredibly clever" Sharon to develop an outstanding advertising copy presentation, winning the attention of Toronto's top advertising agency in the city. Within days, Sharon landed a job there. Taking a deep breath, Marilyn planned to ease back into normalcy, devoting herself to her small children and husband Bob.

Weeks later, Marilyn got a strange phone call from Sharon's new roommate.

"Sharon isn't getting out of bed. She doesn't talk. She isn't going to work. I don't know what to do. But I do know I want her out of here."

Marilyn consulted her husband, Bob. What should she do? Bob urged her to bring her sister back to the house. Sharon was very fond of Bob, and Marilyn hoped he might work his magic, along with a therapist, to get the girl back on her feet. First, Bob and Marilyn wanted to know the circumstances that had impelled Sharon to behave in such an eccentric manner?

"What's the problem, Sharon?" What's holding you up?" Bob asked.

"I can't help it. I'm in love with Minerva's boyfriend."

"Do you mean your former roommate in Chicago?" Marilyn inquired.

"Yes, he's adorable, I love him deeply," Sharon sighed.

"How well did you know your roommate's boyfriend?" Bob asked. "Not very well, but when he carried my bags down on the day I left for Toronto, I knew he was the one. I should get back there right now."

"Just rest up Sharon, and let's talk about this another day when you're feeling better," Bob concluded.

They decided the situation was over their heads, and needed a doctor's evaluation. Sharon resisted seeing a psychiatrist, but trusting Bob, she followed up on the appointment.

The psychiatrist called later, and spoke to Marilyn.

"There's nothing wrong with Sharon. She's lonely, that's all. Just a lonely girl, who needs love and attention. She's better off with you and your husband in a secure, loving home."

"Sharon snowed the doctor, entirely," Marilyn confided to me. "How was it possible?" The idea of taking care of Sharon in her present state along with her four children, including the nursing baby, must have been overwhelming.

Sharon decided not to pursue the psychiatrist's suggestion to remain with the family. Without a conversation or even a note, Sharon packed her bags and left without notice. These early signs of mental illness would follow our sister to Chicago, and once back home, emerge in full expression.

Marilyn's next contact with Sharon was months later at Northwestern Hospital's psychiatric clinic in Chicago, where, after severe acting out behavior that alarmed her roommates, experts finally labeled Sharon's bizarre behavior as schizophrenia.

Once Sharon left our sister's home and returned to Chicago, her life became unwound. Once she landed on my doorstep, the task ahead was trying to understand Sharon as much as possible to make up for the years we had no contact.

When Sharon lived with us in our Portland home for that short period before her mental hospitalization, she left boxes of journals detailing episodes from a failing life in Chicago: jobs lost, roommates departed, friends scattered, lovers gone, all leaving traces of heartbreak and misfortune. I soon learned why I persisted. I became hooked on her care.

Even from a young age, Sharon was a faithful journal writer. Once it was clear she couldn't be alone in Chicago, it made sense to have her personal effects mailed to my home. Two weeks after she landed with me, boxes of journals arrived—twelve heavy containers.

On a cold February afternoon, two months after I had sorted most of Sharon's clothes and personal effects, I tentatively opened a box and pulled out what looked like an early diary. The words haunted me. On the pages, she's a teenager, light and bright, bursting with enthusiasm. Girlish, innocent items: dates and parties, school activities, brother Dave's educational and sports achievements, "Maman's unseemly behavior," Daddy's outbursts. The content could have been mine. Yet, not a word about the married daughters, Nanette and Marilyn, both having fled to safer ground.

Picking up another journal, I could tell by the shift in handwriting and content that Sharon was not doing well. In her mid-twenties, my sister's words seemed halting, angry, vindictive, and self-rejecting. Two startling entries gave me information that should not have been mine to read. Sharon, a devout Catholic, follower of Christ, my sweet, innocent sister, reported two illegal abortions, one year apart, from the same underground medical provider.

I couldn't go on. I felt like a miserable intruder shuffling around with a loved one's deepest, most cherished—and lost—parts. Having just completed a doctoral dissertation on abortion, based on interviews with dozens of college students, I presumed that anyone with an unplanned/unwanted pregnancy felt only relief and even gratitude that their travail was over. After the abortion, the woman would pick up the pieces and move on.

Not so with Sharon. Her grief and anger erupted over the pages. I found myself anguished, weeping for her bitter loneliness in taking that step without family support. Sharon's plight opened my heart to both her and the many thousands of women who, perhaps years later, agonized over their abortion choice.

Maybe Sharon had premonitions about her mental state. Having children to care for would have been impossible. Or her relationships were too unstable, short term or unloving, and that, she believed, merited a pregnancy termination. Having met one of her young men before her breakdown, I found it surprising how casually, even indifferently, he treated her. He seemed unwilling to commit, but Sharon was now a practicing alcoholic. Her drinking, I later surmised, was a form of self-medication. Her boyfriend at the time, a recovering alcoholic, had been a devotee of the Twelve-Step Program for years and stayed temperate. He knew Sharon would be a poor fit for maintaining lifelong sobriety.

I wish I had salvaged more precious memories locked in those journals, but our parents' strong admonitions about privacy, even secrecy, prevented me from opening another page. A few days after my discovery, I asked Sharon what she wanted me to do with the 12 boxes of her diaries.

"Nanette, get rid of them," she replied. "I never want to see them again. Never again. Don't talk to me about them."

I burned the entire batch—all twelve—in our basement recreation room fireplace with five of our children as witnesses.

* * *

Voices! Voices! Voices!

Living with Sharon, I quickly realized the voices were her most intense and disabling symptom. Interminable sounds of fury, rage, insults, curses, and tirades, always damning the sufferer into submission—my sister experienced an unending diatribe throughout her adult life. Despite extensive therapy, Sharon remained convinced that the auditory hallucinations were as real as you and I. Sometimes, more real. They seemed to control her every move. Certainly, they crippled her ability to think coherently or enjoy her life.

"I can't talk now, Nanette," she would say, grimacing and shaking her head. "They're shouting too much, too much."

Sharon's reaction to her voices happened frequently, and although I was aware of her inner torment, I didn't know what I could do about it. I perceived her throat moving as she tried to answer the voices' charges, but a death-like mask quickly settled on her face as she withered under their abuse.

I felt the backlash of her agony, a force that threatened to push me into deep waters, drowning in her misery. I struggled to stay in control of my reactions. I didn't want to accelerate her anguish or fall victim to her illness.

When I shared private sessions with Sharon's counselors, I learned that the voices occur when people misinterpret their inner talk as coming from an outside source. I always took notes during these sessions to better understand Sharon's condition.

"Schizophrenic hallucinations, whether auditory or visual, are meaningful to the person experiencing them," said one empathetic counselor. "Sharon's voices may be of someone she knows, someone or something she fears. These voices are often critical, vulgar, or abusive, blaming her for past behavior. You notice Sharon's voices when she refuses to pay attention to you, but the voices are *more* intense when she's alone."

After further conversations with several sympathetic therapists, I discovered that Sharon's *voices* had evolved over the years.

"At first Sharon complained she heard the shrieks of enraged infants, then nasty toddlers hissing their complaints, and after that, pre-school age brats determined to get attention," the counselor explained. "As she ages, the voices keep shifting; a few years ago, misbehaving school children took over. What followed was worse: a babble of what she calls the 'terrible teens' with their vulgar street language. Eventually, the voices morphed into less abusive but always critical and directive young adults.

"In the last few years, the sounds have had a static-like quality, buzzing, droning like a radio signal from a great distance, but burning her brain and ears with obscene sounds. We try our best to soothe her with medication, but no matter what drug she's on, we can't dispel those dreadful voices she hears."

When Sharon first lived with me, I fought the voices, trying to persuade her to pay attention to her environment, to me, her sister, and to my children.

"I am right next to you, Sharon," I pleaded. "Please look at me; pay attention to your nieces and nephews. Talk to us. We're all here for you."

Her abject look and sharp breath intake could be clues to leaving her alone.

Eventually, I realized she faced those menacing apparitions by herself. Why not join in?

"So, Sharon, what are they saying? Can you tell me?"

Her usual response: "Not now. Just leave me alone."

Occasionally, Sharon gave me brief hints about their presence.

"They're mad today," she told me. "Really angry. They won't shut up. I feel like pounding my head against the wall. I can never get rid of them."

Most of the time, she gave me a vigorous shake of her head as if to say: Lay off. This is my purgatory, not yours.

Sadly, we often sat in silence, me helpless, as Sharon's face turned scarlet as insult after insult lashed her with their cruel power.

But Sharon was wrong. I, too, had been thrown into the same relentless purgatory, and I couldn't find any possible way to pull out of it.

CHAPTER TWENTY-FOUR

More Serious Symptoms

I reflected more than once on Sharon's ironing episode years ago. I quickly rationalized that episode as Sharon's angry reaction to feeling cornered. Dad had insisted she spend the last days of her carefree college vacation looking after my children and me in Washington, D.C. She was apparently in no mood for that assignment. However, what I observed after her Portland arrival was much more severe. I faced the terrible truth that Sharon must have been manifesting psychotic symptoms for many years.

After I found an apartment for Sharon, we visited almost daily for those first months in Portland and at least twice a week for years. This time with her allowed me to witness her mental state at its best—but also its worst—when a psychotic episode turned Sharon into a person I did not know.

Learning to distance myself from Sharon's erratic behavior, I decided to make a list of observed symptomatic behaviors in the belief I could better prepare myself to be a more compassionate witness and helper. Perhaps I feared for my sanity, as well.

Tuning out of our interaction was likely due to narcolepsy, a sleeping disorder, which Sharon claimed she'd had since the onset of her mental illness. Another possible explanation: Sharon's stress level was at high alert every moment, generating inner turmoil and exhaustion.

In addition to narcolepsy, Sharon experienced withdrawal, lack of motivation, inability to express emotions, lack of self-care, abnormal fears, disorganized speech or silence, substance abuse, relationship problems, and auditory hallucinations. Updated Diagnostic and Statistical Manual versions provide an expanded version of these symptoms and others.

Withdrawal and reclusive behavior hardly characterized our growing-up years. As children, we had chores, were polite, considered other people's feelings, and admonished to avoid disordered speech or behavior. Even being funny or silly around adults was forbidden. My father demanded that we act responsibly and predictably, which was his daily mantra.

My mother schooled us carefully to smile at all adults, regardless of who they were. Our parents believed in smiles; their three daughters praised for their exemplary public behavior. Our mother invariably cooed her greetings in a street or store encounter with a neighbor or acquaintance, never relaxing the toothy smile. Gossip about these same people would wait until the evening when she would unpeel their characters with our father. It was harmless gossip, they claimed.

How unprepared we were when Sharon, in her mid-twenties, began to *withdraw* from us—all of us. She shut off the phone and refused to open her door for my brother and me when we planned to meet her after traveling long distances.

I learned to haunt her various Chicago apartments, planting my children strategically to greet Sharon when she slipped in or out of the building for a trip to a Lake Michigan beach in summer or a grocery store in winter. Surprise! Being clever sleuths, we rarely missed seeing her on our four or five visits to the area in 1961. Once we encountered her, Sharon acted cordial, welcoming us to the "Windy City" from our Minnesota home.

Yet, each successive year, when our family made the trek to Northside Chicago to visit Sharon, her behavior became increasingly aberrant, disconnected, and problematic. She no longer kept her room clean. Her clothes appeared unwashed and had a rank smell. Often, she failed to eat regular meals. By 1963, her roommates told us she had stayed away for long periods, and they had no idea where she went. They suspected that after she lost her last job, she survived by stealing food from the local delicatessen, despite receiving regular checks from our dad. Sometime that winter, our father intervened and forcibly put Sharon into the nearest psychiatric department.

Before that intervention, many of our trips to Sharon's apartment were often fruitless. Why didn't I give up then? Why didn't I turn around and go home? Forget these impossible Sharon chases.

I couldn't abandon her. I remember receiving loving advice from an older relative.

"Let it go, Nanette. She's wearing you out. You deserve a life."

But she was my sister, my baby sister. She needed my help. What else could I do? That was my thinking. But once Dad placed her in care, the entire family thought the matter was under control: mental health restored. Sharon continued in Chicago, jobless, alone, depending on Dad for monthly checks. I pursued my own goals of a happy marriage, multiple children, and the grand pursuit of a Ph.D.

* * *

A secret I never shared begins with my adolescent vow about my mother. Financial, social, and emotional dependence on her husband severely limited her freedom, and lost inside the suburban vacuity and party crowd, my mother succumbed to severe alcohol addiction.

After all, her favorite brother, Clarence, didn't stop his heavy drinking until his oldest daughter, Patricia, died in a flaming airline crash over Brazil while a stewardess for Pan American Airlines. A horrifying day for all of us, and prolonged grief for Clarence and his family, as they never found Patricia's body in the impenetrable, cannibal-infested jungle.

My vow then: I must live a radically different life. I must be educated. I must earn my own funds, have my own friends, and be independent of family obligations.

When Sharon later entered my life, my vow doubled. Now I must lead a second life. Sharon's brilliance and perseverance in higher education, I will do.

The children she would not have, I will have. Unlike Sharon, I will not suffer the ravages of mental illness.

I will have a joyous life lived in self-awareness and truth.

* * *

As I reflect on Sharon's severe signs of mental illness, *withdrawal* seemed to be only the beginning. Sharon's symptoms leaped upward during her time with me, choking off the faintest remnants of sanity and leading to more life-inhibiting conduct.

Take *narcolepsy*, which immobilized my sister. This condition of short, frequent, and uncontrolled lapses into sleep entails blacking out multiple times over a day. I observed this often when I was out with her. Sharon insisted her condition started at the same time as her mental illness, but I noticed over time that slipping into unconsciousness appeared to be stress related. Often our conversations had a halting, unfinished quality during our twice-weekly dinners out. And nearly every public encounter contributed to Sharon's anxiety.

"It's good to see you, Nanette. I've wanted to check out that movie... Her words trailed off into silence.

"I know you'll love this one, Sharon," I replied a few minutes later. "It has great reviews." Instead of an answer, I realized Sharon had dozed off again after the first few words.

I continued, fully intending to offer *The New York Times* movie review and hoping my words would somehow sink into her shut-down brain.

Another symptom, Sharon's *lack of self-care,* afflicted me far more than it did her. Once an impeccable dresser, she took it in stride when her clothes had missing buttons, holes, safety pins in visible places and too-long pants dragging on the ground—such disarray, even with newer garments. I felt particularly sad about special occasions like dining in downtown restaurants. My stomach invariably lurched when I met my unwashed, uncombed, bedraggled sister looking spacey and unkempt. Who was this imposter who forced his way into my sister, using her as an agent for its nefarious doings?

Once I humorously mentioned to Sharon the discrepancy between her younger, clothes-hungry self, where ample credit cards from Daddy allowed for a trendy wardrobe, and the person today who cared little about her appearance. Sharon never took reproaches, however slight, with a favorable reception.

"You're violating my privacy, Nanette," she said through gritted teeth. "You make me feel contemptible, and you're ruining my evening."

She swung around rapidly to return to her room. Where did all those words come from? I chased after her, gently quieted her down, and quickly proceeded to the restaurant.

I spent half of the evening at the elegant Benson Hotel mollifying my outraged, deranged sister, assuring her she was a beautiful version of herself and dearly loved by all who knew her. I knew then I must never tell Sharon her appearance was outlandish or out of order. It was a wrong note for my sensitive sister.

Once the waitress adjusted to Sharon's uncommon look, we ate a superb salmon dinner with gusto. The waitress smothered a few chuckles in response to Sharon's extravagant praise of the accomplished harpist featured in the restaurant. What started as a disaster turned out to be a huge success. But I could never predict the outcomes.

Abnormal fears periodically haunted Sharon. After I located a low-rent apartment reserved for the disabled and close to my downtown teaching job, we met once or twice a week. I felt Sharon appreciated the frequent contact and phone calls, even though she didn't know about my life and the pressures I confronted.

A few months after she moved in, she tearfully confided that she was due for a "housing inspection." Managers of public housing apartments made frequent inspections to ensure the residents were not using drugs, damaging the property, or committing other violations. Such inspections topped the list of Sharon's worst nightmares.

"A Gestapo strategy of control," she told me. "I feel helpless." The checkups were unpredictable, making it impossible for me to be there for support.

Quarterly, the hard knock on her door meant at least two male strangers tromped into her tiny studio apartment and rummaged in the minuscule kitchen, cramped bathroom, and cluttered living room/bedroom. They ripped off the blue-taped, curled-up newspaper photos plastered over the walls. They also took note of the greasy stove, smelly refrigerator, and two days of garbage under the sink. Sunk again.

"You fail to meet the minimum health and cleanliness standards," the landlord rasped harshly. "Make the necessary corrections, or you'll be evicted."

Sometimes, Sharon dashed out of her apartment after the inspection to go on one of her extended runs, disappearing to places I couldn't imagine. Sometimes, she ignored the requirements, hoping no one would notice. The eviction notice could stay on the door for weeks, untended. At one particularly humiliating moment, Sharon, winded after climbing four flights to her room, discovered a new batch of inspectors had taken over her apartment. They tore off the carefully framed prints I bought her under the outrageous rule that "walls can have no marks of any kind to pass the housing inspection." Her tortured screams sent both men scurrying quickly down the stairs to secure Sharon's rapid removal.

Rather than launch a search for a new apartment, I decided to throw myself on the landlord's mercy, pleading to give Sharon another chance. I hired two students to clean up and, with their help, saved my emotionally battered sister from exile—at least that time.

I learned that *disorganized speech* or *silence* affects many people with mental illness, especially if they are off their medications. In Sharon's case, even when she took her regular anti-psychotic pills, the conversation boiled down to the minimum.

"Yes, I like that," she'd say. "No, that makes me sick." Or "I'd like to see that movie." She could also banter occasionally.

"You're a sight for sore eyes," she'd exclaim, or "Who would vote for that clown?"

Sometimes, she was even willing to share a recent letter from our folks. Sharon always seemed to have updated news.

"Your Dad got a bad cold on the Mediterranean cruise. He was knocked out once we got home, spending an entire week in bed to recuperate, and still running a low fever," our mother wrote.

Such volubility, followed by silence, and again, I stepped into her verbal vacuum, but only reluctantly. Why did I always feel like someone had dumped a bucket of ice water on me when Sharon vacated?

At one point, after a particularly extended psychotic period, Sharon's counselor advised me to have her committed to the state hospital. When faced with three court psychiatrists, my sister followed a now-familiar pattern. Expressing socially appropriate speech for a few sentences, she impressed the court with her sane replies to their questions.

But when pressed, she raged against me.

"You're the poorest excuse of a sister I've ever known," she shouted, turning on me. "Who the hell do you think you are, anyway? This sham trial is your doing."

She spat the worst invectives at me that I've since managed to block out of my memory. She didn't spare the courtroom and other prosecutorial figures either. Forcibly resisting her captors, Sharon was dragged from the courtroom, bellowing incoherently, and continued a litany of insults and curses that reverberated down the hallway. How was that flailing, insane person my gentle sister?

I was unprepared for the post-proceedings period when I felt numb and had a sense of futility in the face of so many of Sharon's distressing and often bizarre behaviors. I suppose I should have felt shame and humiliation by a family member's public display of madness. Instead, I was surprised to feel gratitude and relief because Sharon could obtain help. Eventually, Sharon received intervention in Portland for her tortuous disease.

Once treated and released from this mental hospital visit, Sharon returned to her apartment, and our life together resumed what I hoped would be an ordinary course. I was frequently disappointed.

Why didn't I recognize Sharon's problem with *substance abuse*, considering our mother's long struggle? Unfortunately, I was in complete denial. We invariably celebrated our gatherings with one or two cocktails, wine, or cordials. While I realize now that Sharon's staggering to and from the ladies' room deserved my attention, I stayed in blissful oblivion during those times.

Some occasions, though, yanked me out of my disbelief that Sharon had a drinking problem. What woke me up was a memorable visit with Portland cousins, who enjoyed far more than sipping. Serious drinking began promptly at 6:00 p.m. and continued for two hours *before* dinner. At 7:00 p.m., Sharon was speechless. By 7:30 p.m., she was no longer able to walk by herself. At 8:00 p.m., dinner serving time, my sister fainted dead away at the table and, when moved, started vomiting and screaming hysterically.

After I cleaned her up, the glazed-eyed cousins took only a few minutes to hustle us out the door. I burned with a hot, hard flame. Where were their hearts? What about some compassion? I put a halt to future happy hours with both Sharon and those cousins. As for Sharon, was it possible the medications she took interacted negatively with the alcohol?

*Relationship problem*s prowled on the edge of every one of Sharon's human connections: roommates, friends, lovers, and even family members. Her mental illness blocked out sustained interaction with others. She became quarrelsome. She lacked compassion. She appeared insensitive to anyone's efforts to reach out to her. She fixated on an issue or event, becoming enraged if you disagreed. Perhaps worse, Sharon acted impassive in the face of others' troubles. I think of Yeats, "the center cannot hold," when I reflect on Sharon's tragic losses.

Initially, Sharon resisted living in Portland, insisting she wanted to return to Chicago. My presence nearby mollified some of her terrors. After five years, she claimed the city as her own, embracing the downtown with its array of restaurant choices. I felt such overwhelming gratitude that Sharon managed to "settle down" (still Dad's favorite words), symptoms and all. What a different story from when I initially brought her to my Portland home before I moved her into treatment. Despite my work and plans for her future, my sister's worst demons surfaced, destroying her hard-won efforts to achieve normalcy.

CHAPTER TWENTY-FIVE

The Mummy Vision

D uring one of the more tumultuous periods with Sharon in the early 1980s, I found myself unmoored: fatigued, and without inspiration. My friend, Patricia, recommended a spiritual transformation to shake me out of my downward spiral. Patricia told me that when she received her cancer diagnosis, she sought the relief of a vision quest to figure out what kind of treatments would work most effectively to either cure or at least prolong her life.

My friend had a dependent mother situation, and my tale of woe had been trying to cope with Sharon. As we shared our stories, I admitted to hearing about vision quests but never gave a moment's thought to this idea—too airy-fairy. But I had been feeling more desperate lately and, frankly, depressed. Now, I felt willing to try anything if it worked. She gave me a phone number, and I signed up for the next opening at a nearby Catholic retreat center.

But the agony over Sharon was much worse. Immersed in three days of silence on a vision quest in a monk-like environment—how could I bear it—the no-talking part? But what choice do I have? I can't abide this constant guilt, shame, and sorrow.

After enduring Sharon's two suicide attempts, the long recovery, the police involvement, and the loss of one apartment after another, I can't put up with another minute of Sharon's dramas. I know she can't help it. But as I told my father many times, I've had enough. I can't manage my sister with full-time teaching, family, and weekend commuting. I felt strained beyond belief. Dad had no ears for listening to my complaints.

"You'll work it out. "Don't call me about it again," my father callously told me. What a ruthless guy!

Therapy didn't seem to help an iota; it felt like nothing more than another burden to add to the week's overcrowded agenda. Most counselors just shook their heads, "How did you get involved in this situation in the first place?"

Good question. I wish I had a good answer for why my entire life seems lopsided—no complaints about Portland. I'm working 50 hours a week with students I adore, pulling together a grant to study homeless girls in Portland, and taking Sharon out for dinner and a movie at least once a week, usually twice. But now that the kids are in Bellingham, I have to hustle to get ready for those long commutes every other weekend.

It's hardly a vacation once I'm home. I take a day to rest from the week's exhaustion before reading and organizing weekly lectures while ensuring I have enough time and energy to devote to the family. Monday morning, I'm on I-5 for another five-hour drive. Wow! And all of this commuting because Jim is a dean, and I can't get a sociology job while he has that position. "I'll be headed for an early grave," to use Mom's favorite expression. Did I ever imagine my life could be so chaotic?

This afternoon I'm in my monk's cell, tiny but functional, a shared bathroom down the hall. It's our period for contemplation to access our vision. I'm one of the few attendees without a vision yet. Nothing, it's been only a blank, and this is my last chance. Why haven't I had a single guiding image? I've asked God to show me the way out of my dilemma and answer my prayer: "What can I do about Sharon?"

Yesterday, Fr. Skegan's three short homilies stressed the significance of turning our problems over to God. It sounds like the Al-Anon program I set up at Portland State. I'm grateful to the university administration for allowing me to add a Twelve-Step Program to the student activity list. The best therapeutic sessions I've had over the last years, though, have been John Bradshaw's book and lectures about growing up in an alcoholic family and the significant co-dependency problems. What eye-opening experiences. Bradshaw's message: accept your brokenness; there is no other way to live. Life will be simpler when you come to understand your limitations.

I guess I hadn't accepted my limitations yet. I'm still struggling through the whole morass, thinking I can find a cure for Sharon and that I'm responsible for her. Forever! I'd even looked up a South American shaman whose advocates say cures schizophrenia. Sharon put thumbs down on that idea—fast.

Despite my best efforts, Sharon slipped even deeper into mental illness. First, she refused to visit the family in Bellingham, stopped calling me, and declined my phone calls. She gave up letter writing years ago. What a pity. Sharon had such sweet, literary letters. I always looked forward to reading her news. It seems she gave up reading about this time, complaining that she couldn't see the print and refusing to have her eyes checked. So many losses, it's hard, so hard to accept. And the worst part is that Sharon seems to have given up.

I threw myself on the narrow cot and felt myself crumpling. I was trapped. Sharon and I were both cornered by her illness. Everything looked hopeless.

"Give me strength, God," I implored. I turned my face to the wall in utter abandonment. I was at a dead-end until something tugged at me. I turned over from the blank wall and looked outward.

Within minutes an image appeared, as real as anything I had ever seen. I was facing a standing, open casket, not the kind in which we bury our American dead, but a sarcophagus, a coffin in the shape of a human body, the same type of structure I encountered at the famous Egyptian Museum in Cairo in 1984. This one faced me, and at the time, my heart stopped in disbelief: the strange coffin contained Sharon, bound exactly like a mummy inside the coffin. Her feet and body up to her neck were tightly bound with strips of ancient, yellowing cloth, but her face, with its closed eyes, was uncovered, with white, expressionless, ghost-like features. At the same time, I smelled decay: a horrible smell that made me sick to my stomach. Steady, I thought, do not puke now. I've got to get Sharon out of there.

Was she comatose or even dead? I reached out to revive her, awaken her from her deep sleep, but the casket moved as though it were on a turning platform each time I attempted to touch her. It seemed to have many sides, and Sharon turned and disappeared from my sight each time I reached out. I was shrieking, at least in my imagination, and crying uncontrollably. Sharon, Sharon, come back to me! But the coffin turned once again. Moments later, I realized I could not reach Sharon—could never connect with my sister to cure her. It was not my task, regardless of the guilt and responsibility I carried.

The bell rang. I sat up shivering, staggered to the small washbasin across the room, threw cold water on my face, said a few prayers, and left my cell room shaking from my experience. Time for our last gathering and goodbye—in silence, of course.

The mummy image sank deeply into my unconscious. I still had no specific thoughts about the final meaning of that macabre vision. I never shared it with anyone all those years for fear people would consider me needing a mental hospital bed next to Sharon's. I took some dream classes to deepen my meditation, hoping to clarify the vision, but it never reappeared in dreams or waking time. Over the years, it seemed to evaporate without any conscious control. I always knew it was there, though, inside. I may have learned one lesson: I should stay alive if Sharon is virtually dead; otherwise, we're both gone.

What happened in the weeks and months ahead changed my life.

Shortly after that mystical experience, I felt freer to make personal choices that did not involve Sharon. I began taking spring terms off school to be with my family. I attended more professional conferences, some with my family. Jim and I started taking vacations more often—and most wonderfully, he made frequent visits down to Portland. Above all, I realized I had a life different and separate from Sharon, even as I could love her and pray for her.

How much did the mummy vision shape my self-perception and future choices? Slowly, I began to accept Sharon's mental illness as a permanent condition and not one I could change or alter. I did not stop intervening at the various single-room occupancies, letting one of the staff members inform Sharon I was visiting or taking her out to lunch. Sharon promptly came downstairs and seemed happy to see me. I always had a sense of incongruity when I visited my sister. Sharon's downright refusal to reach out and her apparent happiness when we met in person.

I also maintained contact with Sharon's changing array of counselors, who kept me abreast of Sharon's progress or lack of it. I deliberately dropped the idea that I was the only one keeping Sharon alive and began to see her in a new light: not as a burden but as a joy and a gift.

Much of that positive emotion did not come until an intervention after Jim died. My second husband, Burl, and I found Sharon safe but confined to the state hospital. After she had spent two and one-half years in this facility, I was finally able to rescue Sharon from her plight, take on legal guardianship, and find suitable placements for my mentally ill sister.   Knowing Sharon traveled a different road than my family did not relieve me of my sisterly obligations. I also had to keep in mind that, mentally ill or not, it was, after all, Sharon's journey. So, once again, I stepped forward to embrace my sister and do whatever I could to ease her life.

CHAPTER TWENTY-SIX

A Son's Breakdown

What went very wrong? By 1980, when Michael graduated from high school, our 18-year-old son had a full-on psychotic episode generated from drugs and his first plunge into independence. It was a long story from our first high hopes in moving to Bellingham in 1974 and his complete roust from sanity six years later.

Facing the tyranny of teenage boys with established cliques put our son at a severe disadvantage. By 11th grade, he admitted being torn between two groups, "the stoners," party boys, and the "morally and ethically correct" friends. When he first arrived in Bellingham, Mike tried getting on a constructive track, working out, eating right, biking, lifting weights, and staying off drugs. Even with a permanent move to Bellingham, Mike felt like an outcast. His journal entries report how much he wanted "to fit in and was dying for attention." He was desperate to develop friends, "I wanted to establish myself."

At sixteen, Mike made a concerted effort to turn his life around from "drugs, sex, and rock n' roll," his favorite term for "goofing off," to a dedicated path of fitness and study.

"So, I'm sixteen now and love to ride a bicycle all over the place. The guys at school called me 'biking Mike.'" I really tried to make a physical effort. Throughout high school, I took physical education and even took a bicycle class. I also was one of the best improved in condition: weightlifting and running."

"My grades shot up too. Spring quarter, I was on the honor roll, ran cross-country, had a paper route, and rode eight to ten miles before coming home for dinner. But no one was home for me. I needed attention."

Unlike Tim, who craved independence, made his own decisions, and was free from close parental supervision, Mike needed a steady hand to keep him on track. My commuting from Portland was limited to once a month, overwhelmed with classes, writing, and sister Sharon. With Jim heavily involved in administrative duties by day and writing at night and weekends, the older girls busy with their own lives, and Tim in college, Mike had no one. His journal indicates he decided to be rebellious. "Who would care, anyway?"

Being impatient with Mike as he repeatedly violated house rules was one thing. When I discovered a horde of hard porn magazines under his mattress and bed, that episode entered an entirely new dimension.

A spring day, a good day for our annual clean-up of rooms. I think I told Mike my student helper, Debra, and I would be working downstairs, so he needed to be out of his room by noon. We entered the empty but filthy room with buckets, cleaning supplies, and carpet-cleaning machinery prepared to turn the place spotless. I left Debra and dashed upstairs for more cleaning cloths for the windows when I heard a yelp. "What's going on?" I asked her when I returned.

"Look what I unearthed. Your son has every smut magazine ever made, inside his mattress and under the bed. They're dozens here. This kid better get his act together."

I agreed but felt the blood rush to my head. I couldn't believe this pollution level could be happening in my home. Where would he have found the money to buy so many? How long has this been going on? I knew Mike had issues with girls; he'd never dated in high school. But to resort to this?

We cleared the disgusting stockpile out and left the room with the mattress askew, letting Mike know his trash had been removed.

A roar from downstairs, "someone took away my stuff," making it a good time for me to have a quick talk with Jim about Mike's transgression. Debra and I felt violated by even having to handle the glossy covers with their lurid images as we pushed them into paper grocery sacks for disposal. I believed pornography to be little more than the prelude to violence against women, a kind of validation for men to maintain their dominance by force.

When I told Jim about the incident, he appeared shocked. He lacked any experience with pornography and considered it both profoundly offensive and immoral. Jim encountered Mike as he came charging up the stairs and had some stern words for him. When Tim joined the crowd and found his brother complaining about the disappearance of the slicks, Tim lit into him.

"Mike, that stuff's not only a waste of money but a really dumb thing to do—bringing this crap into the house. What's the matter with you? If I see more of this junk here, I will beat you up myself." Not a sound from Mike, who shrugged his shoulders and returned to straighten out his lopsided mattress. Jim may have added a few footnotes, but his older brother's convictions played a decisive role for Mike. With all of us checking, no more pornography came into the house.

Mike had little success with non-drug using classmates and soon joined the drug crowd for endless "partying." His life spiraling downward, Mike perceived he had no choice except to join the deviants. He yearned for attention from his peers.

Facilitated by prankster older brother Tim, Mike spent much of his senior year drinking beer and smoking pot. Tim conveniently wrote excuses to the high school when Mike was too hungover to attend classes. Tim appeared impervious to this addictive lifestyle, carrying on with college, jobs, and girlfriends. For his brother, Mike, it was a different story.

"I really believed I was on the way to brain damage."

As children, their father frequently blamed the older brother for Mike's misbehavior and accidents. Was Tim's enabling behavior an underhanded way of encouraging Mike's misbehavior? Or, perhaps, Tim was genuinely concerned about his brother's discombobulated lifestyle and wanted to cover his mistakes.

In hindsight, marital separation while the two younger children finished schooling turned out to be a debacle. Once Mike moved into the Bellingham home, Jim proceeded with the same distressful behaviors our son knew from childhood. The tactic learned in infancy appeared to be: ask, keep asking, never stop asking for what you want, and your father will provide.

In the meantime, while Jim was gone all day, Mike had the entire house to storm through with his druggie buddies, vandalizing the home, stealing money and goods, and terrorizing Patti. Mike was often high on pot and liquor, a combination that liberated him from any rudiments of humanity. Jim protested, but it was too late.

I recall the urgency Jim and I felt when we placed Mike in an apartment that summer of his graduation, a chance to share space with a friend. We badly needed to get Mike out of the home. Our son was ecstatic: his place, absolute independence. I realized afterward his rampages occurred when high. Within weeks, he had ripped doors off of his apartment kitchen cupboards, smashing them on the floor and grinding them to pieces. Why couldn't I have recognized that sooner?

Fighting with his roommates resulted in mutual damage and recriminations, giving rise to more serious brawls and further destruction. "Bad trips" required Jim's intervention to avoid sending Mike to prison. We both agreed that, while Mike was acting "crazy," the criminal justice system would not be the answer to his issues and only hasten more episodes. We packed him off to the first of many psychiatric hospitals.

Mike remembers that period. He wrote in his journal.

"After graduation, I was committed to a psychiatric ward and then a halfway house. Just two months after my 18th birthday, I was sent away. I realized I was at a dead end. No goals. Nothing to live for; the beginning of a life that was destined with more dead time, and pretending it was nothing. I couldn't find a way to start feeling better."

After a month's inpatient treatment with a basketful of medications, Mike experienced relatively long periods of stability. He began to recognize that street drugs had unraveled him.

"At this point, I knew drugs were sending me to institutions and places of maladaptation. I was trying to get cleaned up. My Mom tried to get me in the direction of positivity by sending me to a vocational-technical school, studying health careers toward earning a nurse's degree. I also worked part-time in the afternoon as a groundskeeper at the university. Even though I fell asleep in class, it was amazing that I got above-average marks. Maybe it's because the teacher gave me special attention after school."

Mike's work experience offered benefits and detriments. He could see his dad nearly every day, but ex-classmates proved to be a problem.

"I felt happy working at the university where my Dad was. I remember times he would give me rides home. Then, there was another story. I saw former classmates from high school at the university. I felt branded and ashamed because some knew about me as a freak. Paranoia settled in, and I knew I wasn't like them with my drugs. They could go on with life and its goals."

With Mike's low esteem, it didn't take long before old drug buddies appeared, bringing more trouble for Mike. The "nothing works" period, I called it, where the entire family sought to avoid Mike. We were all in lockdown that summer and fall, waiting for the next psychotic outburst. The despairing father saw no recourse except to provide the funds to enable his son's using, a non-solution to his son's addiction.

Frantic to keep Mike out of the home, we entered a cycle that went on for years. Jim paid for damages on one apartment after another, settled his fights, and when landlords refused to rent to this "bizarre kid," Jim brought him home to "sober up" for a time. And between such times, Mike would enter another, different hospital, and each time determine to "get straight." Home remained the default location.

I asked Patti how she endured that period, and she said in an email.

"Michael really went off the rails when he set the back door on fire so his 'friends' could come and go as he liked." It was a terrifying nightmare for a 12-year-old who couldn't leave. I recall wanting to disappear...just have the earth swallow me whole. I didn't want to live for a time. The constant fighting between Mike and Dad was hard. Dad just letting Mike do whatever he wanted wasn't much easier."

After at least two major psychiatric interventions, Mike continued to drift from our home to friends' sofas, into independent apartments, and then cycle back home. Probably a year passed before his destructive behavior finally caught up with him, leading to one of many expulsions from the family nest. We were desperate for a solution, and a short-term one came.

After Tim returned from his five years in the military, he cast about for the right job, one that gave him a living not only for supporting his growing family but also something that appealed to his need for independence and love of the outdoors. With help from the family, he bought a lawn service and, knowing Mike needed structure, hired his kid brother.

Mike enjoyed working, even if he could not hold any job for long. Despite Tim training him with the whip—pushing, shouting, swearing, scolding, but never failing to praise him—Mike managed to hang on for over two years, maintaining his apartment and taking pride in his accomplishments. We felt infinite gratitude for Tim's taking Mike under his wing; it looked like a long-term arrangement. The day Mike walked off the job, leaving Tim disconsolate after all his training, was an intensely sad day for me. Mike could not manage the military-type discipline with his bipolar condition. Again, he recycled into the family nest. We needed another solution: fast.

Taking the term off to work on my research, I enjoyed Sue and her family, her husband Jody, and daughters Carrie and Meghann, who were living with us at the time. The young couple had a paper route while Jody attended college, and our son-in-law became a family favorite. Jim enjoyed spending time with him, a former high school athlete. I remember them chuckling and shouting together as they watched basketball, football, baseball, and when Tim was around, golfing.

The congenial circle of males must have excluded Mike, or at least his dad chose to ignore him at such times.

One spring afternoon, Sue and I heard an explosive sound from outdoors. When we peered out our respective kitchen windows, we saw Mike, his face contorted, his body spewing hatred and rage, slamming on the mailbox at the end of the drive, pushing it flat against the ground. We both cried out, and Jim, working on one of his highly-praised political science textbooks, rushed from his desk in the back bedroom to calm Mike down. Instead of appeasing the overly excited boy, Mike took an aggressive stand, lifting the shovel to strike his dad. Only Tim's intervention saved his father from harm.

Somehow, the incident was forgotten. Denied. And life went on with Mike's outrageous behavior swept under the rug. Also ignored were Patti's efforts to protect herself from further victimization as she shoved the bed and dresser against the door. This situation never surfaced as more evidence of Mike's growing psychosis.

Patti's getaway from Mike involved frequent visits to Sue, now living in Mt. Vernon, about half an hour from Bellingham. She loved being in their family circle with her beloved sister and fun brother-in-law, Jody. "I wanted to be just like him," Patti reported.

But one summer, Jody's friend, Max, showed up to recuperate after a bad auto accident. His reputation as a troublemaker continued in his friend's home, and Max directed his venom against Patti.

"That's when Max began his exhibitionism and later started the abuse. All those weeks, I fled from Mike into what I thought was a safe haven, but Max was grooming me, exposing himself, talking dirty, and providing pornography."

I never fully understood the depth of Patti's anguish until recently, when she disclosed how close she had been to suicide.

"As a child, my niece had been victimized as well, probably around the same age (seven or eight-years old) as I was then, maybe younger; she also had symptoms of an ulcer. She would have meltdowns nearly every night at bedtime. At 17, when I was staying with Sue over that dreadful summer, living in Bellevue with Max, I realized he had cut a hole from the pantry into the shower and was watching me."

At about the same time, Mike confronted the end of his unproductive life in the family when I received an official letter. Mike had told "inappropriate stories" to his niece, who, in second grade, must have thought them funny and passed them on during a "show and tell" period. The teacher, appalled, dashed into the principal's office to give an account of the problem, who promptly reported the incident to the Washington State Child Protection Services. The gist of the letter required that either Mike leave the residence or my granddaughter depart within the next 72 hours. But learning about Mike's abusive behavior with his niece had opened another wound for Patti. Finally, I discovered this was my opportunity to move Mike, once and for all, out of state and, hopefully, out of Patti's presence to preserve any remnants of sanity for her.

"I was a high school sophomore when I heard Mike talking filth to my niece. I couldn't go to school for several days. I was so upset. I had actually repressed the memory of my original abuse [from Mike] at 5."

Patti had suffered through the entire Mike-induced trauma, but the niece's episode gripped her again. I speeded up the effort to get Mike out of the house.

Michael's older sister, Kathy, told us about a great halfway house for dual-diagnosis patients—both substance dependent and mentally ill—near where she was working on her Ph.D. at the University of Texas. That was the destination I had in mind when I told Mike to pack up his things as we would be going to the airport pronto to comply with the stipulated time.

Jim protested but outvoted, he listened to Sue, Patti, and me, who recognized the urgency of stopping this insanity from destroying everyone. Jim's denial and misconceived protection of his disturbed son rose to the fore when Patti told him she had been molested by Mike, "So...these things happen," he said. Nothing more.

Jim wept as Mike left for the airport, their codependency shattered for the time being. Shortly after that episode, Sue and her family left for Michigan, removing herself as Patti's protector and escaping what must have seemed like a haunted house. She also abandoned her grieving father, who, bereft of coping skills for dealing with his severely damaged son, faced the prospect of a broken family again.

Where was I during this grandiose devastation of family bonds? Taking a practical approach, I rushed Mike to the airport, kissed him goodbye, told him I never wanted to see him again until he stopped using, decided to behave himself, and sought to establish whatever order in his life he could muster.

I prayed Katherine could manage the situation and was delighted she connected Mike to the Twelve-Step Program and his new protective living digs.

When Mike called a week later, talking about his fantastic trip, Jim laughed it off as a "good visit with your sister, Kathy," and promised Mike he'd be down soon for a visit. The following summer, on Jim's urging, we drove to Texas to see our two children, Katherine, now a fervent Twelve-Step member, and Mike.

Delighted by Mike's progress, we saw the possibility of a recovered son, free of drugs and alcohol and psychologically stable for the first time in years. Mike had long needed this type of caring community, backed up by his no-nonsense sister, a protective housing situation, and frequent counseling sessions. While humble, his busboy job suited Mike perfectly as he learned interpersonal skills while waiting on tables and interacting with staff. I viewed the circumstances as ideal, a stabilizing condition for Mike as long as Kathy stayed at the university. Jim regarded Mike's circumstances as *temporary*, plotting a course to rescue him, a decision that would evolve into another cycle of Mike's undoing.

With treatment Mike's tender, loving side came out, convincing some family members that Mike was inherently going to be okay. Mike sent us this rare Christmas card one holiday season, revealing his soft side and loving gratitude.

"To the greatest parents anyone could have and the most special couple and Mom and Dad. It's nice to share always in such little time in the small world we live in together."

With such loving messages, Mike's relapses appeared crueler than ever.

CHAPTER TWENTY-SEVEN

Dual Diagnosis

When did we realize that Mike had a severe mental health condition? Initially, we noticed various bizarre symptoms: sleeping all day, shouting abuse to family members and friends, cooking huge meals in the middle of the night, and bringing home unsavory characters he picked up, mostly late-stage addicts. Looking back, Mike refers to his slide into mental illness as "being totally nuts." Of his friends, he journaled, "Those guys just used me for drugs and food."

The symptoms added up, making it imperative that we take Mike to a psychiatrist. We presumed the primary issue was mental illness, hence the psychiatric interventions. But it was more complicated than that. Classically trained mental health providers tended to overlook Mike's deep involvement in alcohol and drug use or wrongly believed it could be medicated out of him.

The out-patient/in-patient circus commenced: my worst encounter with mental aberrations. As a parent, I felt morally, legally, and emotionally responsible for Mike's condition, unlike my sense of sisterly duty to care for Sharon. Juggling two mentally ill relatives, I had to keep my priorities straight. My Bellingham family had to come first. As for Sharon, I spent far too much time and mental energy holding our father responsible for abandoning her. Funny how blaming him gave me occasional relief from the moral burden. I certainly could not point the finger at Sharon for her illness. I felt compelled to blame someone.

Sharon's dreaded diagnosis of schizophrenia did not describe the whole person that was my sister. Although she could be a quiet, withdrawn patient, once on her medications, counselors told me they enjoyed being with Sharon: "She's such a well-mannered, intelligent person, a delight to work with."

Mike's often destructive acting out rendered him a social misfit, neither pleasant nor accommodating. My heart sank. I had that queasy feeling of trying to breathe underwater, stressed out by powerlessness, unable to help my son. Our boy didn't stand a chance of having a happy life.

Once we placed Mike in an outpatient therapy program with a highly-rated psychiatrist, we stood back and waited for him to stabilize. The doctor suggested some possible mental illness diagnoses: obsessive-compulsive disorder, bipolar condition, hyperactivity, sleep disorder, borderline personality, schizoid personality disorder, mood disorder, highly impulsive disturbance, anxiety disorder, or perhaps all of the above.

I was stunned by this inventory of ailments and felt the misery of the multitude of mothers who have lost their children to mental illness. Of course, the missing link at this point was the psychiatrist's failure to recognize Mike's addictions.

"Now, don't worry about Mike. Let me figure out what's going on or if he's only acting out a difficult adolescence," the physician reasoned.

My parents also urged me to "let the doctor do his job. After all, he has the best care money can buy," my Dad said.

But Mike remained obstinate and troublesome. That's when Jim decided to move him out of our home—not to a safe haven with mental health supervision, but into a nearby apartment—to restore family peace.

Eventually, we grasped Mike's dire situation by talking with his siblings and observing his friends. We later learned Michael had a dual diagnosis, alcohol/drug dependency and bipolar illness. We concluded that addiction was the primary diagnosis, which triggered the psychiatric episodes.

I took spring and summer terms off teaching and, over the next two years, found a part-time teaching job at Western Washington University. Time with my family allowed me to spend two afternoons a week attending psychiatric sessions with Jim and Mike. This time away meant neglecting Sharon. I knew she invariably had setbacks when I was not there regularly. What choice did I have?

I resisted the psychiatric intervention, the extended, circular interviews with our stressed-out family, bringing up woeful images of Sharon's fearsome aversion to their bleak and intrusive methods. I resisted exposing Mike twice weekly to the game-like atmosphere played out under the treatment rubric, locking him into a category so dense he could never crawl out. They're so easy with negative labels, these doctors. The psychiatrist recognized my doubts and agreed to see me privately to talk about Mike's "progress."

"I see no progress here, Doctor. I need to see something more positive coming from these sessions. If anything, the sessions create more anxiety for Mike. After a therapy session, he overreacts to everything we say and do. We're not even treating his drug addiction."

"Don't worry, I'll give him stronger medication to override the drugs."

His response left me breathless and ready to move on to another mental health specialist. This one seemed to have no understanding of drug addiction. After our conversation, the psychiatrist shifted tactics, urging us to try making a contract with our troubled son. Here's how that session went.

"Now, Mike, promise your parents you'll keep the curfew, follow house rules, and drive more carefully. This sheet of paper will monitor your behavior from now on. Your behavior is completely under your control, and you will be your own scorekeeper."

"Sure, whatever you say, Doctor. It's just people bug me. I can't stand being bugged, makes me crazy. And the medicines make me sick. I don't want to come here anymore."

The psychiatrist initially deemed Mike's outbursts "extended adolescence," treating it as a benign condition, hence the contract. Not until Mike's repeated episodes of beating up roommates—and being beaten up in return—car accidents and speaking word-salad, the garbled language of the insane, did Dr. Do-Little wake up to the frightening prospect that Mike had a severe psychosis.

I reached out for a diagnosis, enabling Mike to receive his daily cocktail of anti-psychotic meds. Jim and I began a dozen or more years of frantic hand-wringing and mutual blame. I discovered that mental illness is insidious, as it fosters the blame game so familiar from my childhood. I attacked my husband.

"It's your damn fault for being codependent, Jim. You're ruining the boy with the car and money. He needs discipline; to stay on his meds, make some effort to get along with other family members, and stop tearing up his apartments. We can't keep paying out those outrageous damages for his destructive behavior. The boy needs to experience consequences. I'm frankly sick of this whole business!"

Jim snapped back. "Go back to Portland, Nanette. You're not doing any good here. I can handle Mike. Just mind your own business."

The marriage dripped with malice and unhappiness. Jim remained covetous of his sons, resistant to sharing authority. Casting my suggestions into the wind, they swirled like dry leaves, shriveling as they dropped to the ground. Despite the episodic distress we endured with Mike, Jim and I stayed together 50 years until his death, learning from, forgiving, and loving one another.

Still, as parents, we tried everything available, hoping to keep psychiatric and institutional care expenses partially covered with our Washington mental health system and university-based health insurance. We relentlessly pursued 30-day mental hospital stays—14 in total—intensive private and state-supported in-patient facilities, out-patient therapy, medications (especially Lithium), halfway houses, and full-time lock-up with severely disabled inmates—a practice common in our town's mental health system.

We soon dismissed the local in-patient option once we looked at the population of young men, all heavily tranquilized, mainly nodding off in front of a blaring television. Both of us optimistically embraced higher goals for Mike: full recovery from drug and alcohol use, stabilization on anti-psychotic meds, and college or vocational training for self-sufficiency.

Mike careened through his twenties in and out of jobs, community college, mental hospitals, halfway houses, alcohol treatment centers—including a year's participation in an innovative institution in Denton, Texas—a number of live-in girlfriends, a marriage that lasted three weeks, and finally a union with Rita, his wife for five years. Together, they had a son, James, our beloved grandson, a real livewire like his dad.

Mike appeared to be "settling in" to domesticity—or was he? We found most of the maintenance money we sent Rita went to whiskey and pot. Behind in rent, Mike's school and vocational training abandoned, the little family appeared to be sliding into a bottomless pit. Indeed, Mike had lost any moral compass he may have had from his growing-up years.

Out of desperation, I became an avowed follower of the Twelve-Step movement, attending daily meetings for relatives of alcoholics, meeting other family members with similar stories, and slowly feeling stronger and more capable of handling my son. Perhaps, I felt more centered than Jim, despite, or perhaps because of, my double duty with Sharon and Mike, as my husband elected not to follow my lead into the Twelve-Step spiritual program. With a friend, who had a decade in the Twelve-Step program, we devised a plan: an all-or-nothing last-stage-of-this-madness proposal for Mike. Both of us suffering from severe burn-out and facing financial ruin, Jim and I must have a workable program or join the ranks of the lost.

We laid out our do-or-die program, a tough-love scheme. Mike would enter a lockdown public Oregon institution for long-term alcohol and drug addicts and stay until he could remain "clean and sober," I hoped unrealistically, forever. We planned to deny him money, housing, and family support. The consequences would be dire if he decided to relapse or demanded release before completing the program.

Jim reluctantly bought into the program. What else could he do? My husband had no plan, no faith, no hope, and no love. He had burned out on Mike. I felt him closing down in self-preservation, leaving me lonely and unsupported. I stayed with the mantra: we cannot give up on Mike.

I convinced Jim to stop rescuing Mike with money, requiring Mike to face up to his behavior. Now convinced that Mike could not be a good father because of addiction, Rita began divorce proceedings. His siblings had long dropped away, exhausted by his unpredictable and harmful behavior. If Mike could not get his act together with this last and final hospitalization, he would have no one! I delivered the ultimatum standing outside the front door of Mike's apartment. Jim stayed behind, weeping in the car.

The ultimatum included our decision of no communication during his incarceration. We never answered Mike's calls; his appeals fell on closed ears. Alone, forced to tackle the reality of his life—that substance abuse has unraveled his existence—Mike began his slow turnaround into sobriety.

You can see we were desperate, all of us: his wife, his mother, and his long-suffering father. Our reasoning seemed logical, given the circumstances. I did not hesitate to move forward with this stark solution. Nor do I have any regrets now. The outcome turned out as my supportive friend and I prayerfully predicted.

But what if this scheme had fallen flat? What if he refused to stop drinking and drugging, and self-willed, stopped taking his medicine? Do we throw this negligent, addictive, out-of-control person into the scrap heap? Probably not. I'm sure I would have continued my tormented, maternal nagging. Jim and I would have been forced to stop the financial hemorrhaging, paying for private therapies and institutions. Mike would have been more and more on his own. Surely a miserable, ever lonelier life would have awaited him.

CHAPTER TWENTY-EIGHT

Miracles Happen

At one juncture of Mike's veil of tears, and before he entered a lockdown, dual-diagnosis facility, I reached a point of no return with his drinking and drugging. For the first time in his life, I felt hopeless. "I'm ready to give up on this kid. His father and I have done all we can to get him on track, but he's doing nothing but running through our retirement funds. I can't hang out here forever, hoping he'll get his act together."

What parent would not share my lament when their child has lost his way?

DISPLACED

Entrenched in sadness,
Compounded feelings constrict her
As she envisions the lost boy.
His pouring out of Soul in wailful deprivations.

Lack of harmony
Devoid of joy,
Loss of balance,
Deprived of safety,
Erosion of trust,
Dragging in worry,
Depleted of completion,
Uncertain of the future.

She seeks the alone one,
Tangled in delusions,
Forgetting his way,
Paralyzed with fear,
Marching willfully into danger.
Sinking into the fog of despair.

Can no one save this lost son
A wanderer,
Who seeks freedom in misguided pathways?

Early retirement from Portland State and an invitation to study homeless girls in Sydney, Australia, opened new vistas, and I decided to move toward them, temporarily moving away from home. I felt fully justified in abandoning Mike, who had broken every agreement, we, his exhausted parents, had ever made with him about staying clean and sober, getting a job, and caring for his wife and baby.

Finishing my homeless girl report for the Australian Home Office that following summer at home in Bellingham, I was rewarded with another university offer, this time in South Australia, examining the mothers of homeless girls through the auspices of counseling offices in Flinders.

Most of the findings were discouraging; girls left for good reasons—abuse, neglect, disorganized households with unrelated men shuffling in and out, and a general assumption among the mothers in these working-class families that "kids can manage on their own, get jobs, or something." Having interviewed girls in these circumstances, I calculated that most seemed too young, unskilled, and vulnerable to be on their own. Most, it turned out, had little trust or love for their mothers.

When I arrived at Southern Cross University to study the homeless girls' mothers, I discovered the university was a distance away from the city and knew I would need friends and social distractions from the relative isolation. After a few months of reaching out to friendly Aussie women, I had a vibrant social life. My new pals wanted me to experience a full range of Australian activities. Fun outings in my temporary home filled some lonely hours without my family.

"Let's take Nanette to that psychic, Bette, she's great, said one." Another piped up, "I got this job because of her." "She sees into your soul," commented another. It looked like a fun afternoon, a ride out of town, lunch, and woo-woo time.

I retained my skepticism, unsure if such guidance would work for any of my unresolved issues, but I muttered, "Sure, let's go."

We pulled into a dirt driveway next to a small, typical Australian bungalow with dense foliage in the front garden. Not so promising. But my friends' enthusiasm was infectious. All aboard, I thought, as we walked around to the back, Bette's client entrance and her beauteous garden.

My turn. I handed Bette my silk scarf and a bracelet so she could "read my energy."

"Nanette, I have someone here. Her name is Alice. Do you know a person named Alice?" I felt as though I were fainting. How could she know that? "Yes, it's my mother." I don't know any other Alice."

"There's a lot of static here, but her voice has a husky quality. Do you remember that, as well?" "Yes, it's unmistakable," I responded.

"Well, Alice has a message for you she keeps repeating. 'Don't give up on Mike; don't give up on Mike.' What do you think she means here?" I was unprepared to bring up the long struggle I've had with my son and just said something to the effect of: "unfinished business back home." Bette nodded and went on to the next woman.

When I returned home in July, I went to Portland and invited Mike to be baptized by my favorite priest.

"No church for me, Mom. That's not my spiritual life."

"OK. Are you willing to let me baptize you? I will need a witness, and that's it."

I set 29-year-old Mike flat on his back on what I imagine now was a massage table. I planned to pray over him and then administer the sacrament. As I poured the droplets of water on his forehead and dried his skin, the sun shone through the window directly on the table's surface. The witness gasped, and I stared. The uncanny part is that it formed a perfect golden cross over Mike's body. The Holy Spirit comes in diverse forms, I found.

When I told Mike what was going on, he seemed unsurprised, as though he'd been waiting for a sign a long time. That incident must have occurred before he had experienced the lockdown institution and made what I thought was a final commitment to be clean and sober. From then on, I would bend every effort to facilitate his survival.

CHAPTER TWENTY-NINE

Bend With the Wind

I wish I could say Mike's life measurably eased up at this time with troubles forgotten. Such was not the case. Michael must now dance to a different, unforgiving tune, the county mental health system. I doggedly looked for housing, always those limited to dual-diagnosis clients: recovering alcoholics/ addicts and the mentally ill. His continued instability, reflected in frequent run-ins with residents, minor rule-breaking, and failure to attend counseling appointments, brought another ultimatum. The system laid it on the line: any further trespassing of the rules meant he would lose his housing and disability checks.

Mike's options shrunk. He made the right choice: he claimed housing and monthly disability checks were more critical than his distorted idea of "freedom." We felt pleased to have the mental health system back up.

Mike remained in Portland, visiting Bellingham only rarely, once to honor his dad, who died in August 2002 after suffering four years from strokes and heart failure. Mike had also made short visits to see his brother, Tim, and his sisters, trying to heal his divisive relationships. We found a lawyer to assist Mike in obtaining Social Security disability. Unable to cope with visits home, Mike began missing buses and trains, leaving his meds in Portland, and exhibiting anxiety attacks. By 2008, home trips tapered off to zero.

Fast forward to 2015. Mike moved into an Oregon county-subsidized apartment with his son, James. Unable to self-maintain, he suffered from a life-threatening illness and severe malnutrition. James managed to get his dad into an intensive care unit—just in time. Here, he languished for weeks since finding him a safe place required months of sustained intervention.

Back from the hospital, Mike needed new digs. Our housing search, limited to affordable housing through the mental health county office, uncovered few viable choices. Those fortunate enough to have adequate placements tended to stay in place. We hesitated to put Mike in independent housing again and needed family counseling to help emancipate Mike from his untenable situation in the now-ruined apartment.

A few weeks later, we were assigned a counselor, Roy, who competently sorted matters out, arranging for an all-afternoon family meeting with his new client and family. The counselor sought to determine Mike's expressed needs and the kind of support to back him up if he lived in independent housing. The counselor asked,

"Mike, can you get along by yourself in a furnished studio apartment in town? You understand you can't bring in other people to live there unless they're on the lease. And you may be on your own for cooking, laundry, and cleaning up your place."

Mike nodded his head vigorously in favor, weary of living in his grossly damaged and rent-unpaid apartment, the landlady on his case daily, trying to push him into vacating the premises. Mike and his trail of ex-roommates could be likened to a wrecking crew, with rooms stripped to the bare walls, carpets in shreds, and plumbing unusable.

Turning to family members, Roy inquired,

"Do you think Michael can live successfully in independent housing? And more importantly, who can support Mike to reduce the risk of his relapsing or failing to follow housing regulations?"

A few present—ex-wife, Rita, son James, and Michael's sister Kathy spoke up, asserting their intentions to visit regularly and help Mike cook meals, take care of laundry, pay his bills, and whatever he needed. I recognized the signs. No one wanted to put Mike into a confining group home situation. Mike will do fine, just fine, once he has a new placement.

I perceived the direction this meeting was going. Mike would have another start-up, except my second husband, Burl, and I will be the point persons to salvage him after he nose-dives and crashes. From my experience working with Sharon, I'm learning that independent living is the less expensive route for the state compared with more intensive supervision in foster care or a mental health facility. But the emotional and financial costs to the patient and family caregivers can be steep. And I know this now. Many mentally ill persons cannot survive, much less thrive, without mental health supervised housing.

I knew Michael's pattern so well now. Living alone, he becomes tortured by loneliness. He has time now for regrets about his former drinking, drugging, and inability to hold a job. He suffers anguish over disappointing his late father, who had such high (and unrealistic) expectations for him. He feels sad that he has had a series of fallings-out with his older and much-loved brother, Tim. When living independently, he reached out for a roommate, a batch of roommates, all of whom took advantage of him.

Over the years, I heard stories about Mike getting beaten up, his food eaten by the passing parade of strangers, and his ex-wife's shirttail relatives who moved in and out of his apartments on a regular basis. As a result, he lost the apartment, unable to maintain himself. The saddest part: he has had no idea how to break the pattern.

Burl and I, living hours away, were discounted as steady support. His sister, Katherine, living in Olympia, two hours away, would not be available for emergency assistance. That left his son, James, in his early 20s, to carry the ball. Having tried this kind of support and finding it unworkable, I shuddered: too little assistance, the wrong type of help. His son, experimenting with alcohol and pot, had shown he wouldn't be a good influence on his father's addictions. Rita, who had remarried, was unlikely to be available to perform caregiving duties for Mike. Despite her avowals to give Mike daily care, her priorities would be for the new husband, not Mike.

The long afternoon meeting with my son droned on. Overcome by what I perceived as a lost cause—getting Mike the supportive framework that would allow him to survive—I collapsed into tears. I felt the crushing weight of futility if I didn't state my case fervently; give an account of the years of efforts I have undergone with family members to keep Mike intact; the number of institutions, therapies, counseling sessions, twelve-step programs, and pain we have felt when confronted with "nothing works."

Roy looked at me sympathetically. I'm hysterical and cannot stop sobbing.

"Nanette, you appear troubled. What's your take on Mike's housing situation?"

"I can't abandon him now," I cried out to Roy and my family members.

"Please, let's find him appropriate housing that allows him to live successfully, accommodates his disability, and gives him self-esteem and hope. Isn't this the least we can do for my son? I can't believe the system could be so heartless as to consign Michael, now 53 years old, to still another round of illness and failure and to ignore my exhaustion trying, again and again, to make it right for him."

A long moment of silence. I apologized for my outburst, but it had results. Different stories emerged about Mike's distresses and catastrophes. Everyone wanted the best for Mike. The consensus shifted. The group agreed Mike needed more assistance in daily living, including scheduled medications, meals, laundry, bill payments, and planned activities. Independent living, the group concurred, was clearly out of reach.

Mike was mainly silent, listening to us, awed at the care and attention directed his way. No longer rebellious, Mike went along with the decision to move him into a county group home two miles from Rita's place. The meeting concluded with plans for regular counseling and recommendations for how we could assist Mike through the period before securing a group home. Rita, greatly underestimated, acted as the chief caregiver for Mike during this interim period.

Months later, group housing accomplished, Mike flourished, gained weight, perhaps too much weight. He loved Maribel, the house mother, her superb cooking, and making friends among the other four residents. He cherished weekly dinners with Rita and her new husband, relished James' guitar music-making, and, blissfully for Burl and me, stayed calm and centered—even during visits to Bellingham with his son.

By May 2018, at age 56, Mike demonstrated a new kind of quality: leadership. What I believed was that Mike had finally come into his own with an offer for peer leadership training. For a moment, I experienced joy, trusting that an amazing transformation from that dismal family meeting in Roy's office three years ago had occurred. Mike could make it as an independent person.

Michael even brought me his completed memoir, all 200 pages of his recollections over a lifetime. We instantly liked the fitting title: "Inventory of a Bi-Polar Addict." Like his parents and sisters, Sue and Patti, Mike had taken up writing, although not at the same level as other family members. But my optimism about his progress soon evaporated.

Once again, Mike regressed when his foster home closed down, and he was placed once again in independent living after treatment for mania. He had overcome a psychotic break in December 2021 with a self-directed period in the hospital, followed by a highly supportive rehabilitation team. His apartment complex, once a structured environment with supervision for the mentally ill residents, had been converted to regular clients. Mike remained the sole disabled person in his set of units, and without anyone in charge or frequent contact with the mental health system, lost his way.

When my son resisted treatment and publicly acted out his severe symptoms, he attracted predators who abused him. During a recent episode, he experienced intruders who broke into his apartment, assaulted him, stole his phone, Social Security, health, food stamps, bank, and other access cards, vandalized his home, and ended up with his eviction. After a period of homelessness, when he developed pneumonia and flu, he went into detox. His body was incapable of surviving in the homeless condition. He currently awaits resettlement in a different location, but the trauma associated with this event has broken his sense of safety and security.

What I have learned in the process of loving my son is to "bend with the wind"—the favorite saying of my yoga teacher. I have accepted this bleak prospect of his psychotic episodes and will undoubtedly continue to feel anxious about my son. I recognize how easily he slips back into the ravages of psychosis. Who knows the reason? Has mental health support failed? It appears that it has. And does my son willfully remove himself from care, believing he is no longer mentally ill? His hallucinations suggest both situations may be at play.

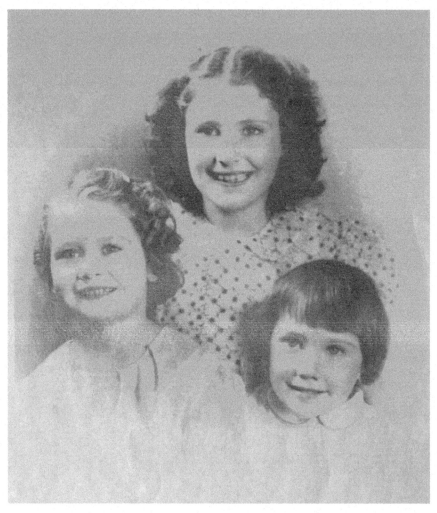

Three sisters (left to right) Marilyn, Nanette, and Sharon, 1938

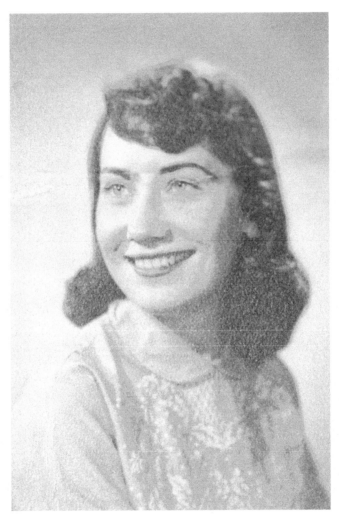

Sharon's graduation from New Trier High School, 1954

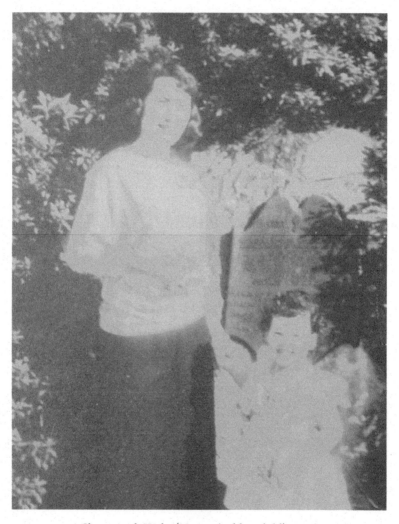

Sharon with Kathy (Nanette's oldest child), 1956

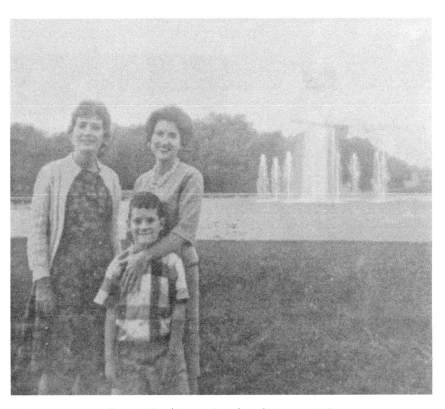

Sharon, Tim (Nanette's son), and Nanette, 1961

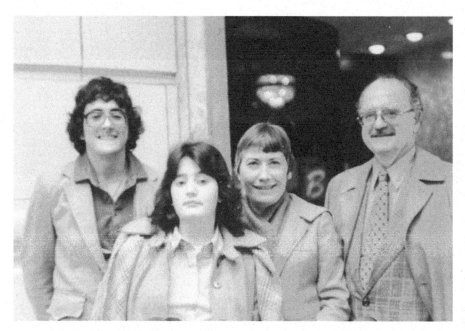

Disneyland with (left to right), Mike, Patti, Sharon, and Jim, 1978

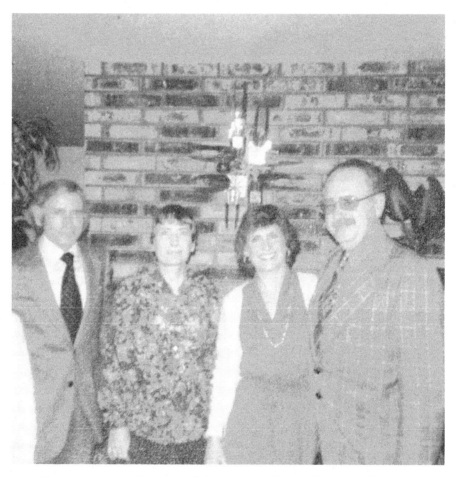

Christmas gathering (left to right), family friend, Sharon, Nanette, and Jim, 1982

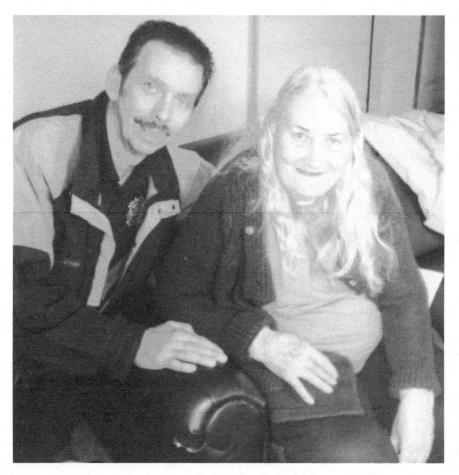

Sharon in a transition house with Dan, Katherine's husband, 2009

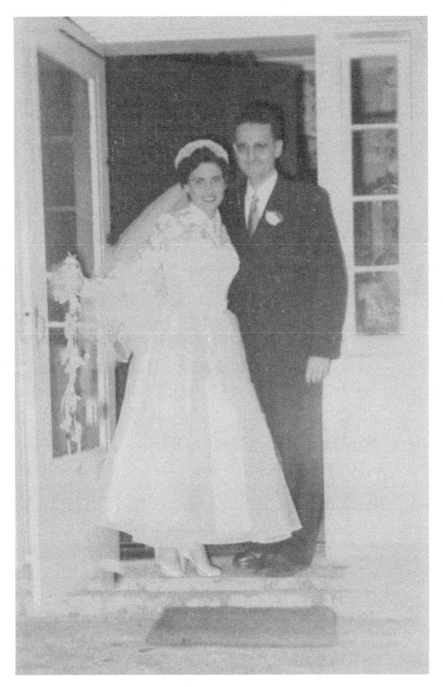

Wedding Day, 1952

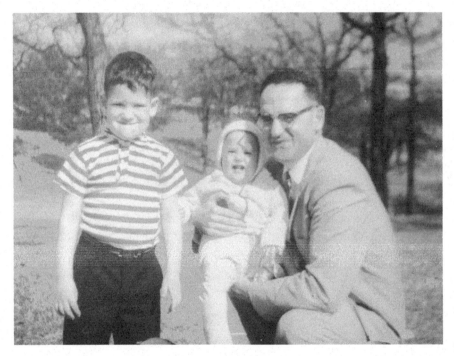

Tim, Mike, and Jim, 1962

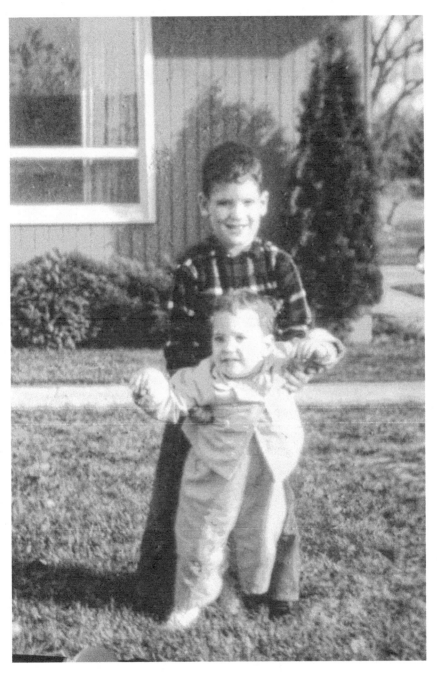

Older brother Tim and Mikey, 1963

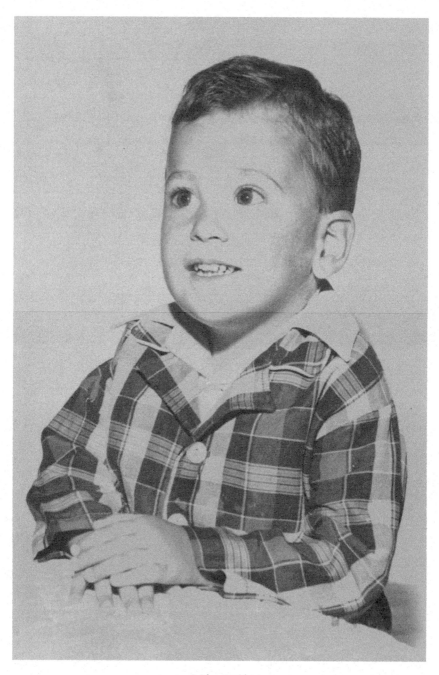

Mike, 1964

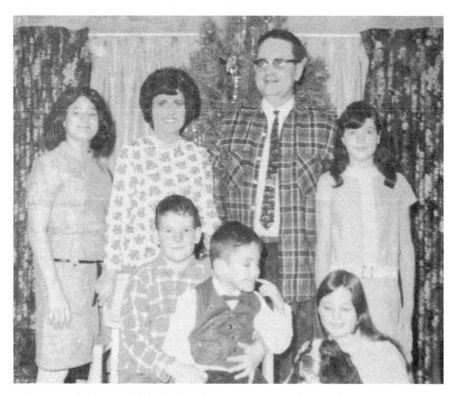

(back row, left to right) Kathy, Nanette, Jim, and Susie (front row,
left to right), Timmy, Mikey, Liddy, and family dog,1964

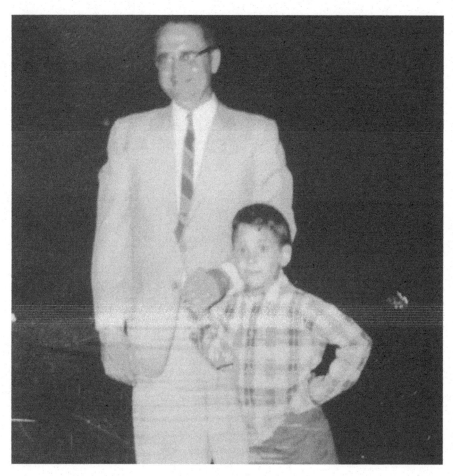

Mike and his dad, 1968

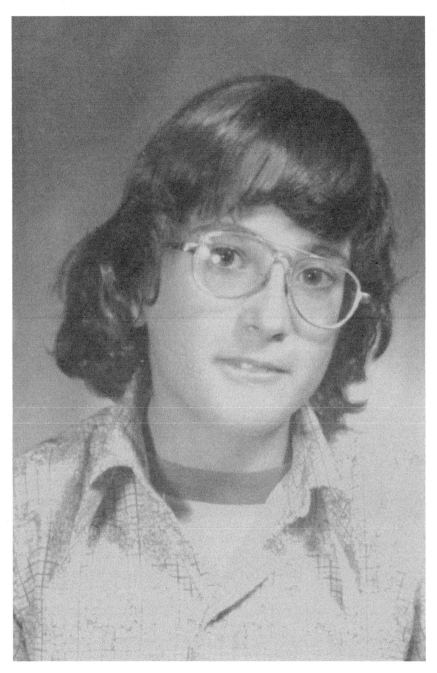

Mike, 1971

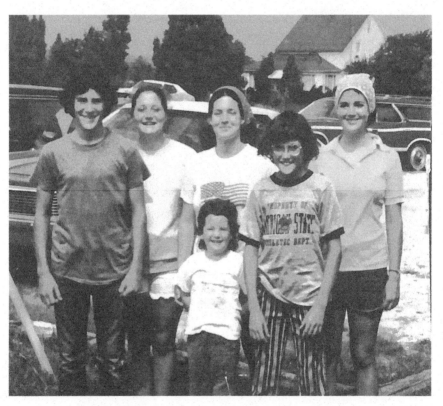

All my children (back row, left to right), Tim, Liddy, Kathy,
and Sue (front row) Patti and Mikey, 1972

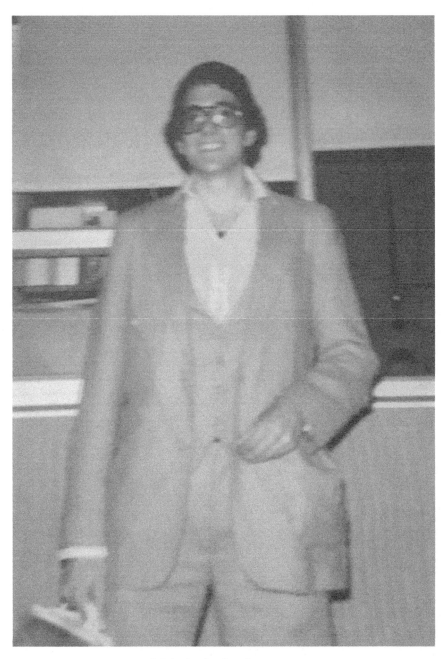

Mike's high school graduation, 1980

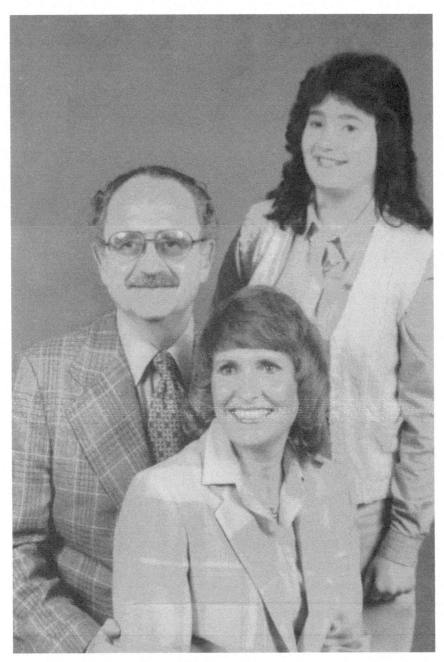

Jim, Nanette, and daughter, Patti, 1981

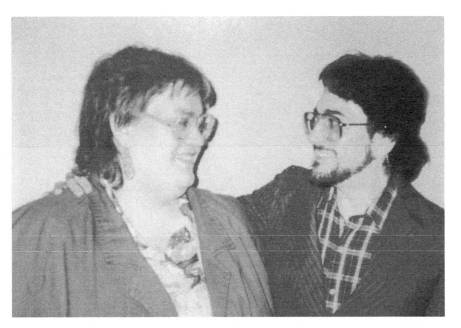

Michael and his new bride, Rita, 1990

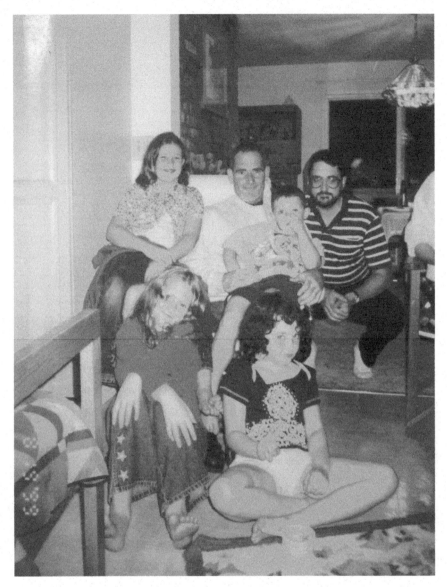

(back row, left to right) Tim's daughter, Rebecca, Tim, Tim's son, Timmy, and Mike. (front row, left to right), Tim's daughter, Rachael, and Katherine's daughter, Eleanor Grace, about 1995

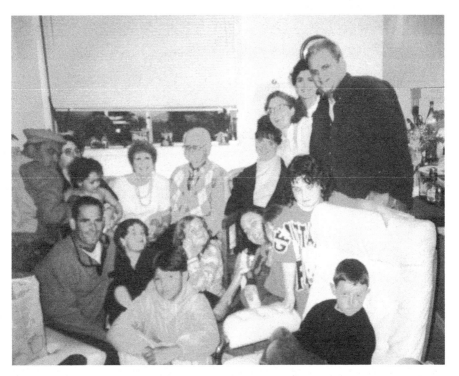

Happy family gathering, about 1997

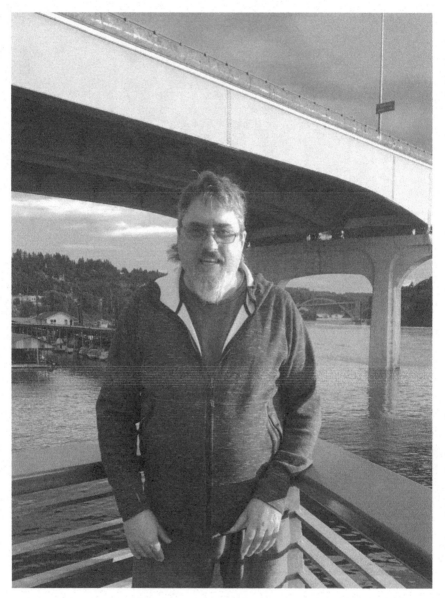

Mike, clear-eyed and confident, in a local park, 2018

Part Three

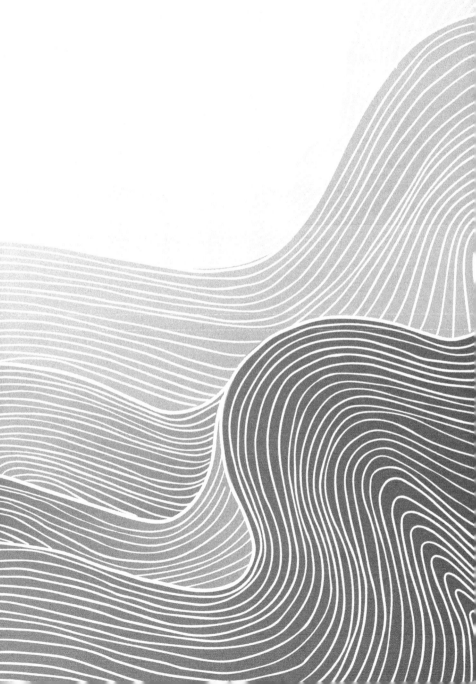

CHAPTER THIRTY

Caught in the Cuckoo's Nest

After weeks of trying to locate Sharon, our sister Marilyn miraculously found her at a state hospital. Marilyn urged me to visit our sister after all these years she was lost to us. Appalled, I found she had spent the last two and one-half years institutionalized without any responsible staff—after all that prolonged time—making any effort to contact the family.

After extensive talks with Sharon and hearing her side of the story and the reports from the hospital counselors and staff, a few of the patients, and my own sleuthing, here's what I could make out of those lost years I was separated from her.

Sharon went from very bad to disastrous: no more counseling, case management, or even contacts with the mental health system. Her mental disabilities increased, and she found her only solace in isolation. The run-down lodgings where she had formerly lived had a prison-like atmosphere. Staff was there to maintain control and little else.

After years of neglect, Sharon had become delusional, unaware of herself or her surroundings. Lacking a shower, adequate wash basin or towels, Sharon abandoned self-care and was beset with vermin: lice, bedbugs, fleas, and I shudder at what other insects assailed her. Eventually, the hermit was rescued when the housing staff identified the foul odor from Sharon's room—of course, she wouldn't open her door—and they called the police.

The rescue squad came but left immediately to put on their complete personal protective equipment (PPE) after confronting her appearance, swollen with bug bites and comatose. Without medication for months or even years, she was hospitalized for her medical needs and then transferred to the state hospital for a lengthy mental health rehabilitation.

Sharon initially did not rehabilitate well. She resisted assistance, missed meals, dodged staff requests, and acted out her most severe schizophrenic symptoms: hallucinating, shouting, and resisting help. Isolation remained her only friend. Even after months of care, Sharon showed little interest in ward activities or mingling with other patients. Staff recognized that Sharon despised the institutional routines and could barely tolerate being cooped up in a bedroom with four or five other women, "all equally insane," Sharon said at one group meeting.

Staff told me Sharon slipped out of an open door on one warm summer day and probably said to another patient, "I need some fresh air." It took three staff persons to bring my resistant sister back up the two flights of stairs and into the ward. I understood the situation well because Sharon had never been easy to corral. Not only did she have a moment of blissful freedom, but she stumbled on a half-consumed cigarette and happily puffed away on the contraband when the security guard caught up with her.

Despite her aloofness and withdrawal, the ward administrator, Evelyn, said that once stabilized on her medications, Sharon behaved politely and showed a willingness to accommodate. She always said "thank you" to the servers and smiled at the patients sharing her dining table, although she often had little to say. As I recall, Evelyn told me,

"We all apologize about Sharon's extensive hold here. We inquired if Sharon wanted us to contact family, but she always vetoed the idea. Not only did Sharon say "no," but a vigorous and loud "NO!" Add to that, the psychiatrist required guardianship. This meant that Sharon could not be released without a legal guardian approved by the state. Since she refused to have anyone she didn't know "control" her, we were at a loss as how to proceed. She was adamant about staying put rather than submitting herself to more legalese. Our hands were tied."

Years ago, when Sharon first left our home under police protection and was placed in care, a hospital therapist inquired if I was willing to serve as Sharon's guardian. After reflecting on my split life with my teaching job in Portland and my family life in Bellingham, five hours away, I had to say "no." I could not accept the terrible responsibility of Sharon with her failure to stay on her meds, her frequent relapses, and her dreadful resistance to help.

Moreover, the Court wanted me to pick up all the costs of care "befitting a loving family member," said one court administrator. Taking over Sharon's mental health care was one thing. But taking charge of Sharon's monetary needs seemed over the top. I felt justified in rejecting guardianship at the time, but after seeing Sharon in her unfortunate predicament, I realize I perhaps made a profound mistake.

Sometimes, when I think about Sharon, I can only drum up my list of mistakes, shortcomings, and absences. The state hospital refused to reveal Sharon's location because we lacked the appropriate "documentation." The state required "full consent" by the deranged patient—who could not give consent—meaning that severely mentally ill persons without a guardian have no family access. I suspect Marilyn must have hired a private detective to uncover Sharon's whereabouts. All my efforts ended in red tape without access to my sister.

Sharon spent two and half years cramped in a small room with four other mentally ill women. She was ready for me to step in as legal guardian and release her from this detestable institution. Still, I had strong misgivings about serving as legal guardian for my sister. Was I taking away her sovereignty as a human being? With a mere signature, I take charge: determine where she lives, how she lives, what she eats, and even who her roommates will be. These decisions I eventually took on for her. Yet, I felt unfit for the job. Who was I to dictate the various medications required to still the voices, allowing her to live and converse normally? What kind of sister snatches away a person's autonomy, meeting the court with dry eyes, stating the facts of my sister's lifelong schizophrenia that rendered her wholly unfit to live alone, care for herself, or make sound decisions? Once I faced these issues and considered the unbearable consequences of not accepting this responsibility, I fully committed myself to Sharon's care.

My talent for nagging the system finally paid off. Sharon was assigned to a well-appointed, state-operated mental health adult home, a transitional setting between the hospital and a standard assisted living facility. It seemed incredible. At last, we found a vibrant environment where Sharon could genuinely flourish. Still, I was wary. Burl and I took a very long look at the situation before deciding to move Sharon. We were overjoyed when we discovered the facility had a strong reputation for positive patient outcomes.

It struck me later why I tried so desperately for so many years to keep Sharon happy, healthy, and as content as possible once I accepted the reality that my father never planned to assist her. All the effort I put in trying to save our mother from herself—all lost. Perhaps with Sharon, I could be redeemed from not saving my mother. Especially after our mother's premature death, I sensed an urgency to protect my sister.

After my experience with my husband, Jim, in various nursing homes, I learned to be cautious about institutions. We decided to try Sharon's new placement and planned to visit often. Sharon has needed an advocate for a long time, poor girl. I had left her in the lurch for too long.

I blamed myself for letting Sharon sink this low, extremely broken down in mind, body, and spirit. But I also knew I had grown weary of constantly bailing her out, rescuing her repeatedly. Part of that time, I was too preoccupied with Jim's last illness and death to assist her. I promised myself I'd do better this time. Now that I realized what I could do for Sharon, I let go of my hand-wringing.

What a shock to see Sharon after all these years. Unbelievable! She'd been in this lockdown ward for such a long time. I always thought mental hospitals existed to stabilize patients with brief recovery periods. Why hadn't anyone called me? I knew that at one time, my name was on their lists of approved contacts or whatever that list is supposed to denote. None of the family knew where she'd been for years. I figured this prolonged stay could be grounds for litigation with this damnable outfit, but I was happy we finally found her. I had no energy to pursue what could take years with few results for embattled patients.

Before her mental illness, Sharon was a fashion plate, always meticulous. I remember her having daily showers and maybe two or three in the hot weather. She always wore impeccable clothes, had her hair newly cut and curled, and was ready for what our Mother called the "Easter Parade." But now, in the institution, she had food-splotched clothes that didn't fit, dirt under her fingernails, foul body odor, and her breath! It nearly blew me away. Her face had taken on a grey pallor—the same color as these dreary walls.

No sunlight seemed to come through the dirty, barred windows. The saddest part: Sharon's hair, unwashed, uncut, hung limply over her face. She looked like she'd given up.

This ward must have been the "last stand" zone. She was not the only one who looked pathetic. All the patients had a haggard, lost look. They seemed absent from their own lives. It's as though they'd confronted the noonday demon, and the beast would not let go. What an insidious curse, this mental illness.

While I was angry that we didn't hear a word from the mental health system for all this time, I had a sense of gratitude that Sharon at least had a roof over her head, and their care prevented her from injuring herself again. Sharon needed a secure program for many years. Let's hope the next facility does the job.

Even as we extricated her, the system inflicted one more insult. Sharon could not retrieve the gifts we'd given her over the last few months, while she was waiting for an available bed at the next facility. Her possessions had disappeared: radio gone, clothes missing in the communal laundry, and personal hygiene items vanished. I said to Burl,

"Even monks, who turn over all their worldly goods to the order, are allowed to have some personal property."

Privation fits the no-privacy surveillance program they run here. How can anyone be a person, a conscious, aware being, in this dreadful place? Sharon arrived with nothing. Now, she leaves with nothing. I felt angry over the entire situation but vowed that with the family's help, I would set Sharon up in a supportive situation.

CHAPTER THIRTY-ONE

Almost Safe

After taking wrong turns for the last 40 minutes, Burl and I finally located the mystery building where Sharon would live—we hoped for years. The southeast Portland neighborhood looked shabby with its odd collection of apartments, single homes, and empty lots—not exactly what we prayed for. We pulled into a small parking lot of a slightly upgraded, post-World War II, grey stucco tenement house—Sharon's new home. We rang the doorbell and waited for the staff to open the door. It all takes time. We fidgeted and wondered what was in store.

Once in the main lounge, we took another look. A large all-purpose room held tables with games, recent magazines, low-volume television, and dining tables set for four next to the open kitchen. We were about to be more surprised: fresh, clean aromas—absent the urine-soaked carpet stench of some of Sharon's former dwellings. Other plus signs: appetizing food aromas, busy residents moving freely about, and a smiling staff welcoming us to "Transition House."

Sharon rediscovered her intentional voice: song, speech, and silence. Burl and I found her wide grin and marvelous, husky chuckle—so remindful of my mother—completely heartwarming. We visited every few months, sometimes more often, with Burl bringing his guitar and vocal talents along with song hand-outs, a gig he does so well in various assisted living and nursing home facilities in Bellingham.

Sharon knew the old standards by heart: swing tunes, folk melodies, romantic refrains, and many original arrangements. We belted our lilting tunes to the gallery along with staff, a few other residents, and sometimes, James, my grandson.

Sharon could be finicky in her musical choices, "no," on whiny-voiced Westerns, "yes," on Glen Miller, Tommy Dorsey, and Duke Ellington. She and Burl regaled an eager audience with stories of the big "hits," humming familiar tunes with Sharon laughing at every hint of nostalgia. No longer shy, my sister welcomed the residents and staff who joined our singing group. I felt touched by these people, not only the dedicated staff but also the patients, their tragic stories, and their plucky survival.

"No more Nurse Ratched for me, Nanette."

Sharon's reference was her impression of the dictatorial supervision at a state hospital, epitomized by the infamous Nurse Ratched in the film "One Flew Over the Cuckoo's Nest." Sharon's modus operandi, if I can call it that, has been to avoid control, resist control, and fight control. As a close student of Ayn Rand, Sharon flooded her young adult mind with Rand's highly individualistic perspective, expressed in novelistic form. Rand's "take no prisoners" slogans buzzed brightly for her.

"The smallest minority on earth is the individual. Those who deny individual rights cannot claim to be defenders of minorities." But Rand forgot about our collective well-being.

Here's another one: "The question isn't who is going to let me; it's who is going to stop me."

No middle ground here: "There are two sides to every issue: one side is right, and the other is wrong, but the middle is always evil."

Making compromises hardly reflected Sharon's values. Her tenure at this new facility still did not reflect who this person truly was: a competitor, a lone wolf, a take-charge type. But now, a space opened for her to test her capacity for control.

Let's take Sharon's domino playing, hardly a pastime. She played to win and win always. During her time at Transition House, Sharon never lost a game, never took pity on her opponents, and never stopped playing until she'd demolished the opposition. How reminiscent of our ever-competitive father.

Sharon transformed into a leader. She radiated a vibrant presence at Transition House. In month four of her stay, Burl and I walked into the main hall and flagged a resident. Other residents looked up to her and followed her daily actions and activities.

"Hi Mack, where can I find Sharon?"

"She's playing cards in the East Lounge. Before that, she was in group but plans to have another domino game she's set up after dinner once you folks leave."

Sharon controlled the domino scene, knew where they were located, put them away after use, placing each tile neatly in the box. Passive no longer about the "inane" television shows once endured in her former captive incarnation, her choices prevailed. Surprisingly, everyone agreed. Concert music, public television, and classic film DVDs resonated in the common room anytime Sharon moved to watch. Small fry victories, you might think, but Sharon felt satisfied with such achievements. I only needed to see the benign expression on her face.

A resident let me know about Sharon's newly found status.

"Sharon's the smartest person in here. She knows what's going on. I've learned a lot. Did you know she was once a top writer for an encyclopedia?"

Sharon set her own boundaries: too much coziness, too many people around, overstaying our visit, new resident arrival, requiring intensive staff attention or noise, she took a stand. "I'm tired now," and disappeared into her room. We never followed. Sharon needed her privacy. Even with a single roommate, she claimed alone time. I observed the roommate, Penny Ann, who took a hint, murmured "hello," gathered her purse, left the room, and silence ensued. Sharon finally had charge of her domain.

Self-care turned out to be a different matter. Sharon showed little regard for "dressing up," her clothes frequently littered with food stains and crumbs. I bought her batches of attractive outfits, slacks, and tops. Our sister Marilyn sent pajamas, robes, and sweaters. Why did everything look like the bottom-of-the-barrel items at a garage sale? Hair, nails, and clothes all had an unkempt look. Sharon shrugged it off with a who-cares-what-it-looks-like attitude. I spoke to the staff.

"Could we try to sort out Sharon's appearance? She looks neglected. My sister and I keep bringing in toiletries, a comb and brush set, and cute, upscale clothes, but she throws everything in the closet. What gives here?"

"Yes, we're having conversations with Sharon. She hides her dirty clothes and refuses to let the laundry people into her room to pick them up. She doesn't want her clothes 'mingling' with the other residents. We only have 17 residents, and half are women. Her clothes are washed only with the women's. We've reached a dead end. Any chance you could wash them at your house and bring the clean clothes back?"

"Impossible," I insisted. The distance is too great. We've traveled nearly six hours to get here today with heavy traffic on I-5. What other options do you have?"

"Private laundry service."

"I'll take it and pay the difference."

Once we made this minor change from collective to private, Sharon took a moderate interest in her new clothes. At least she began wearing new outfits that suggested she "gets it." These clothes were hers and hers alone, never shared, even in the washing. I also pleaded with the staff to motivate Sharon to see a dentist, encourage her to try out a new hairdo, and push her into trying the fun outings offered by the House: a symphony, a walk in the park, and a zoo trip.

The young, strikingly attractive administrator, Debra, fresh out of graduate school, appealed to our understanding of what staff must deal with.

"Sharon refuses all our recommendations about leaving the building, Nanette. The psychiatrist indicates she's exhibiting a classic pattern of agoraphobia and only feels safe indoors. Of course, we have to take her to the specialist occasionally—such as last week when she was coughing so badly—but that requires a special attendant. In addition, she only consents to go when wearing a blindfold and crouching in the back seat during the ride. I'm sorry, but if she has another emergency, we must use a sedative to avoid a panic attack. It looks like dentistry and shopping are out of the question."

Wouldn't Sharon be happier with new gleaming teeth? Luxuriating in a salon with fresh hairdos? Going out to plays, the park, the zoo? All the other residents jumped at the chance to get away for a while.

It was not to be. I finally realized Sharon's outer persona might have altered, but her fears of displacement and abandonment paralyzed her.

The staff and I encountered another roadblock: Sharon's increasing weight. Again, I talked with compassionate Debra, who offered several reasons for the growing obesity.

"Over the last few years, Sharon has experienced serious nutritional deficits. During her stay at the hospital, she often refused nourishing food in favor of bread or sweets. She's having a grand old time with our great gourmet kitchen. We've got the best chefs in the system."

"Another consideration, your sister may be self-comforting with the extra portions. At least, that's what her counselors think. We typically don't interfere with residents' food choices unless there's a problem. Of course, we monitor calories to ensure proper weight management."

She continued explaining why Sharon had weight gain and seriously swollen legs.

"Another culprit is the new medication, Abilify. Do you notice how much more alert and alive Sharon has been over the last month? It's the new drug she's taking. We find that some of our residents are extra hungry with this medication until their metabolism settles down after a few months. We're still exploring how to manage the problem. Right now, Sharon's leg swelling calls for treatment. I'm sorry to put you in this position, but you'll have to sign the papers for us to limit her food intake and allow medical intervention."

Eventually, Sharon achieved the necessary balance with Metformin, which, when taken along with Abilify, helped to regulate her blood sugar and stabilize her weight. Too late for Sharon. Her overweight condition failed to lessen, contributing to a pre-diabetic state, severe leg inflammation, and chronic back problems. As her watchdog, she called me on the carpet.

"You don't know what you're doing. You're not my boss! I'm eating completely normally. I'm tired of everyone trying to fix me. Damn it, they've cut back on my food. I'm hungry all the time."

Could this be a slight exaggeration, as I watched Sharon eating heartily, including today's small wedge of chocolate cream pie? I commiserated with her, reminding her of all our dear Mom's regular diets, but Sharon stayed firm. She blamed me for interfering in one of her main pleasures, second helpings. And, of course, for asserting my authority over her will.

After a few years of being the top domino player, an established music connoisseur, and a board game specialist, the agency gave Sharon notice she must leave this haven and move on to another facility, "Comfort Corners." I soon learned that this new facility was a good-enough staffed adult family home for mentally ill seniors but lacked the rich resources of Transition House.

I fought for weeks to keep Sharon in her existing living arrangement, arguing by phone and letter with state bureaucrats about her precarious mental state and their years-long neglect of this incapacitated woman. I pleaded with them to provide the in-house medical and psychiatric services that previously contributed to Sharon's remarkable recovery. In desperation, I even hurled insults

244 · NANETTE J. DAVIS, PH.D.

at a couple of obstinate administrators who did little more than cite their rules, always *their* rules. As legal guardian, I received Sharon's eviction notice, which read something like this.

"Sharon will be moved to Comfort Corners, an assisted living facility, in two weeks, where she can fully access community-based physicians, psychiatric care, and physical therapy. This new situation is the best we can do with our limited resources. After all, we let Sharon stay an extra year at Transition House, bearing in mind her difficult case. As we informed you over the phone, Transition House is restricted to persons immediately released from the state hospital or other institution."

I felt like someone had just run an ice cube down my spine.

Of course, Sharon never benefitted from preventative community-based mental health care or other so-called accessible programs since she remained unwilling to leave her comfort zone to go anywhere. Bureaucrats rarely consider those victimized by incapacitating phobias that prevent sound choices.

After opening herself to new people and activities at Transition House, Sharon closed down again, never fully recovering that secure sense of place. We all did what we could to lighten her spirit and reignite joy. Burl and I continued bringing music; happily, Sharon willingly joined in. Our visits always included gifts: stuffed animals, good, lubricating body creams, and scented soap. Dorothy, a nurse, and facility co-owner with her husband, took charge of seeing that Sharon had a good television hook-up and her favorite DVDs. The nurse even brought in her electric-controlled recliner from home, enabling Sharon to slip on and out of the chair without assistance. Sharon's wan smile was her "thank you."

Sharon lived for three years at Comfort Corners, from ages 74 to 77. Beloved by staff and residents, she struggled with advancing asthma, chronic obstructive pulmonary disorder (COPD), intense back pain, immobility, and a barrage of people, medicines, and treatments I knew she found intrusive. I realized medical matters were serious when Dorothy called with the terrible news.

"Nanette, I'm sorry to be the bearer of bad news, but your sister fell yesterday at the bathroom sink and hit her head. You know how weak her legs are. Worse, she was unconscious for hours, and our house nurse indicated she must have had a serious concussion."

Predictably, Sharon rejected seeing a doctor or psychiatrist. Her physical condition worsened; the depression deepened. Only one option left: hospital treatment that Sharon convinced herself was a "fate worse than death" (one of our mother's pithy phrases). When Sharon was finally taken to a nearby private hospital in 2012 after a life-threatening episode of COPD, she endured relentless panic attacks, rejected treatments, and shut down completely. Yet, the facility rules required that her lung condition receive hospital care unless otherwise determined by the legal guardian. Dorothy told me this story by phone about her efforts to get Sharon to the hospital.

On a freezing January day, the ambulance pulled up to the front door at Comfort Corners to whisk the critically ill patient to one of the local private hospitals. There was a struggle. Sharon refused to go and was sedated. Because I was out of reach in Mexico, my cell phone apparently immobilized, the facility had to take matters into its own hands. As the guardian, I was supposed to consent to medication changes or hospitalization.

I knew Sharon had waited for me to protect her from this latest insult, but time had run out. After two weeks in the hospital, her insanity returned full bore. My suffering sister lost again, described by staff as "raving, hysterical, and unresponsive" to the army of strangers hovering over her bed. Meanwhile, her home facility refused to take her back because of the grave nature of her illness. Only the hospital could manage her pain and symptoms, the administration insisted.

Once I returned from Mexico, I finally made contact with the hospital and facility and signed the necessary papers to release her from the hospital's clutches.

Wounded and dispirited, Sharon returned to Comfort Corners once again. Trying to make amends, I assured my sister that I would never force her to undergo another "tormenting hospital" encounter. Comfort Corners staff signaled their disapproval of Sharon's return because they lacked appropriate staff—and never said aloud—feared the stigma of death should Sharon die in their facility. Sharon stayed, protected by the state's mental health laws.

But I did not give up trying to persuade her to return to the hospital. Persistent, but not pushy—Sharon balked at anything too insistent—I tried to convince her that hospital treatment had some real benefits.

"It can be life-saving," I pleaded, despite Sharon's protests. "You can get better pain medication at the hospital. They can treat your engorged legs and provide physical therapy for your back. You might even be able to walk again. Your living unit at Comfort Corners is an assisted living facility, not a skilled nursing unit. They can't do much except keep you comfortable. And they can't even transfer you into their small nursing ward next door because that's booked up for the foreseeable future, not one bed available."

Sharon's only rejoinder: "I need to be left alone. I'll be all right. Don't worry about me."

I translated her supplication as: "Please, no special attention, as I can't seem to tolerate any more interference in my personal space."

The hospital episode opened Sharon to more than simple protests about unwanted medical care. At one of our visits, the suppressed rage I often experienced in our interactions over the years spilled over into a full-blown angry outburst.

"I've had it with all you people, pushing me around, telling me what to do, where to go, what to eat. Who consults me? You're doing it over my head. And who gives a good damn about me, except when you're around, which isn't too damn much. Where's Dad once he left Portland after a single visit? Where are Marilyn and Dave? Do I exist for them? I have no family. Mom's gone, but she was gone with drink even before she died. I am so fed up with all of you for disappearing after I had my first breakdown in Chicago. You can all go to hell!"

Oh my God, I thought. What gives? What could I say to her? Did she expect me to say or do anything about this dreadful life she's lived? How could I ease her mind? What was there to say? I apologized, as I had done so many times before after Sharon launched a momentary—or more extended—tirade against me at our time together. Not extended episodes, mind you, but I always felt diminished when they occurred.

I can't recall everything I said on this occasion—I know I was shocked, utterly stunned at this outpouring. Naturally, I felt a wave of guilt, hearing these denunciations, recalling the years I visited not at all, especially when caring for Jim. Before that period, I admit my first obligation was to Mike. I couldn't stretch myself any further. But that all sounds like excuses, doesn't it? From Sharon's point of view, we were all failures at loving and caring for her.

After the verbal explosion, Sharon lapsed into silence, staring into space, appearing relieved for letting it all out: her anger, her pent-up feelings, her losses, her emptiness. I stayed through dinner that evening, where her spirits seemed restored. I noticed the high color in her cheeks and her louder-than-usual laugh. She needed to make that statement. I needed to be the witness. It was a harsh lesson for me, simply listening and being with her. I know now that Sharon's outburst was her way of expressing grief for her lost life.

After a year of illness, Sharon rallied the Christmas before her death. December 16 and time for her birthday party. Who could resist it? Burl and I brought special treats: a large, white stuffed bear dressed in holiday garb, sweet-smelling lubricating creams, and cards from all the family. We gathered in the common room for birthday cake, a magnificent three-layer homemade white cake with chocolate icing. As Sharon cut the first slice for her admiring fans and visitors, we heard a heavy knock at the front door. It was the UPS man delivering boxes of birthday gifts from sister Marilyn—just in time. Sharon's luminous smile won everyone's hearts that day as she celebrated her 77th birthday, opening gift after gift after gift.

After Sharon's rescue from her long hospital stay, Burl and I prayed daily that her last years be spent in a good, secure, and loving place. After such an unspeakably difficult and dangerous journey, Sharon surely deserved to be sheltered with care.

I believe she mainly achieved that safe place over the last few years, but only up to a point. Sharon's lifelong struggle with mental illness involved not only degraded housing, lack of comfort, and poor nutrition. More than that, its radical influence unequivocally separated her from almost every measure of adult success: health, wealth, home, family, friends, lifetime job, personal security, and the capacity to make informed choices. Sharon deserved the best, but over the years, she received only the worst that life can deal to anyone.

CHAPTER THIRTY-TWO

Eulogy for Sharon

Background.

After Sharon's death on May 24, 2014, we gathered eight of us in the Portland area who knew and loved Sharon. We held a memorial service in the small chapel of the Omega funeral home two days later. The following steps were cremation and picking up the urn of ashes to hold until we had another memorial with Marilyn and her family on the East Coast in August.

I suspect Sharon's long-drawn-out life—death at 77 years old—was far more prolonged than she wanted. I honor the fact she held to her promise that she would not attempt to take her own life again, that she would wait for the "hand of God" for a natural death. I was dreadfully conflicted. Had I known what unbelievable torments she would experience with her mental disorder, would I have stepped back and allowed her to take a different course? Possibly choose her own time and place of dying? It's difficult for me to say now. I mistakenly didn't question my motives or Catholic values. It always seemed so important to keep my sister alive. Given her fierce independence, she remained a challenging subject for behavior modification. As Frank Sinatra, one of her favorite crooners, sang, "I did it my way." That's the spirit of Sharon we learned to cherish.

The following August, my husband, Burl, and I carried Sharon's ashes to my sister Marilyn's home, where we had a different family gathering with our brother, Dave, and his wife, Ann. Marilyn's son, John, and his family, also joined us as we scattered her ashes in special planting areas at a nearby beach park: an exquisite tribute to a courageous woman.

Here is the eulogy I read at the May 2014 Portland memorial.

* * *

Eulogy for Sharon

Greetings on this special day of honoring Sharon, our beloved sister, and friend. As we gather together, we pay homage to Sharon, a dear lady, a powerful soul, whose earthly life was made so difficult with chronic mental illness from the age of 27 and, in her later years, tortuous physical disabilities.

But Sharon was never about her limitations. She was always a person, more significant, more expansive, and more profound than the mental illness that sometimes held her mind captive, but never her spirit.

I brought Sharon to Portland from her hometown, Chicago, in 1975, and over the years, I loved, appreciated, and honored her spirit. Once stabilized on her medications and nestled in the trying-so-hard Oregon mental health system, Sharon and I had extraordinary moments. Sharon's favorites: occasional plays, good restaurants, weekly movies, especially foreign flicks helped keep us once-detached sisters attached and loving.

Sharon was indomitable. Regardless of her external circumstances—living in dilapidated one-room hotels, homeless, bereft of friends, and often alone without family support—she surmounted every obstacle. Visits were only occasional after I retired from Portland State University, yet we always enjoyed our time together when job and family demands made it possible for me to travel.

I was mainly absent from Sharon's life during the four years I was caregiving for my late husband. Then she slipped out of sight, lost to a system that kept us guessing as to her whereabouts. Sharon did very poorly on her own, we discovered. To stay safe, she locked herself into her dreary single room, free from predators, to be sure, but essentially desolate and abandoned. Somehow, she managed to hold body and soul together, despite the enormous difficulties of daily life, including bug infestation that afflicted her body.

I know now how intensely grueling her situation had become, as cutbacks in mental health funding plunged Sharon and others like her into despair, trusted counselors disappeared, help and hope faded, and life became increasingly unmanageable.

Over the years, the family lost track of Sharon numerous times as she moved from one blighted living condition to another. But we never let her go. We persisted, and during one of her extended periods of no-contact, finally found her in 2009 at the state hospital, reasonably intact and eager—after a protracted two and one-half years—to relocate. When I introduced Burl, whom I had recently married, Sharon looked at him carefully, then glanced at me, and with a big grin, told me what great choices I had made—for both husbands! We all roared with laughter in these otherwise somber sanitarium halls.

Released from the hospital to a transitional facility, Sharon flourished, developed friends, and learned to play games—her domino skills were legendary. She embraced classical and modern music alike and loved the attentive staff. Sharon was kind, constantly extending a warm greeting to anyone seeking her company. She even had "boyfriends," lonely middle-aged men who liked to tell their stories to a listening ear and an open heart. Still, Sharon managed to maintain her cloak of privacy.

Burl and I soon learned Sharon had an ear for melody—she was a veritable songbird. When Burl showed up with his guitar and rich baritone voice, and I with my less polished one, we blended our happy harmony. Sharon laughed in all the right places and delighted in the old standard swing tunes Burl played with such facility.

Sharon resisted the move into Comfort Corners, her final home. She had made good friends and felt so at ease in that first post-hospital setting, geared to reclaim patients who had wandered far from their moorings. In the second facility, she often seemed overwhelmed by new routines, different people, novel activities, and an all-female residential unit. I strongly encouraged staff to invite Sharon into the common room—she preferred staying in her room most of the day, and it took many months before Sharon warmed up to inviting others into her life.

Burl and I visited Sharon three months before her death, and with my grandson, James, we noticed the visible decline. Constant, racking waves of coughing triggered fractures in her back, previously broken in 1976. Her vivacity was lost to breakthrough pain, requiring extraordinary measures of an oxycodone and fentanyl cocktail to provide some semblance of well-being. Walking was hampered by fluid, swelling her legs to enormous proportions. Her lungs were attacked by chronic obstructive pulmonary disorder that eventually took her life.

As Sharon gradually wore down, there were repeated trips to the hospital, a place Sharon feared and hated. On many occasions, I pleaded with the staff to provide care *within* the facility rather than inflict the hospital's impersonal regime.

In her last few weeks, I wrote an order for comfort care, but staff said Sharon's continuous outbursts hampered their efforts. I knew they were expressions of independence and integrity. She refused help over and over, adamant about not wanting to be an invalid or receive special attention. More importantly, I believe the staff lacked the expertise to deal with her numerous maladies. Although I repeatedly urged the administration to call in hospice care those final days, it never happened.

Miraculously, a bed opened up in the facility's nursing unit during the last week of her life, allowing Sharon to finally relax into more intensive care and accept the ministrations of a devoted staff.

Sharon died an independent person. Even in the end, she resisted the nursing staff's efforts to keep her going with oxygen. Oh no, not for Sharon to continue lingering, and who, when nurse Tammy turned her back, ripped off the mask that gave her breath, and chose her moment of death: a final victory!

Sharon taught me some fundamental lessons.

Accept life as it is.

Keep your word.

Be grateful to those who help you.

Be a proud, independent person, regardless of your circumstances.

Smile through your pain and suffering.

My three oldest daughters: Katherine, Susan, and Liddy chose to remember Sharon in her earlier years—by her wit, her beauty, her joy, her love of life—when everyone was young and oh-so-very hopeful. Katherine remembers Sharon's often repeated, hysterically funny (if distorted) phrase—at least for these youngsters—"Hotsy-Totsy, I'm a Nazi," followed by tummy-gripping laughter. Sue recalls the splendid sunny day when Sharon was tasked with taking the children to Mass, but instead, with a giggle, picked them up for joyriding and ice-cream cones.

After hearing of Sharon's demise, Liddy commented, "I remember Sharon as drop dead gorgeous, driving in her shiny, new red Mustang, and proudly parking it in front of our house."

That's the image I'd like us to take away today. Sharon—beautiful and free, no longer lost, surrounded by angels—driving her shiny new red Mustang straight into Heaven and parking it at the front door for eternity.

Elegy for Sharon

Y ou didn't give me enough warning, Sharon, when you slipped so swiftly into those last weeks of dying; softly, they told me—plenty of time left.

But they didn't reckon Sharon's galloping speed down the runway of death and letting go of life's excesses: lungs, intestines, brain, all exuding mucous fluids, repulsive to touch or smell. She was only too happy to release the burden of pain.

And so alone you were, dear sister, without the comfort of family to support your leaving, without the Church's "Jesu, Joy of Man's Desiring," as the goodbye salute for the next lap of the journey, without the grieving mourners surrounding your deathbed. You rejected them all in your hasty retreat. You shut me out of those end-of-life memories and left me hanging. After all our years together, Sharon, you slashed the sisterly cord and took off on your own, leaving me empty-handed: leaving you angry and inconsolable in your unfinished life.

And nothing left for me to hold. Nothing left to hold.

A Final Word

Then and Now. Treatment for mental illness has transformed since my sister was first institutionalized in 1963 and my son in 1980. Today, although limited in practice, recovery programs exist for various mental disorders—schizophrenia, PTSD, bipolar disorder, borderland personality disorder, ADHD, OCD, depression, anxiety, eating disorders, suicide, addictions, and others. Such programs reflect growing knowledge and new intervention tools to help the mentally ill, their families, and their communities.

But our society has barely begun to dig in and confront the unmet needs of millions of Americans with mental illness. In a recent newsletter, the National Alliance for the Mentally Ill announced that we have more than 60 million people, or one out of five, living with mental illness (NAMI Newsletter, October 2022).

A special section of the *Sunday New York Times* (October 16, 2022) painted a doleful picture of the current state of care, especially for the 14 million or so who have severe mental illness, including bipolar disease and schizophrenia, and who cycle in and out of psychiatric hospitals, jails, and homelessness. The NYT report says, that despite our increasing knowledge about mental disorders, "there is still no community mental health system in America." The report also pointed out that political decisions continue to determine whether care exists, what kind of care, and who receives the care.

"Handcuffs, not help," the slogan for Sharon's era, relied on forcible psychiatric intervention, primarily emphasizing medications, but rarely succeeded in convincing the patient to cooperate with the drug regimen. Like my father, who relied on a straitjacket to tie Sharon into treatment, I also depended on punishment: harsh intervention of police action to ensure my sister's eviction from my family home.

I perceived no other choice. Sharon's severely disordered behavior included the inability to relate to other family members, difficulty perceiving reality, failure to handle daily problems, intense outbursts of anger, and bizarre sleeping patterns. These problems were excruciating intrusions on our family peace. Repeated failure to comply with her treatment plan of medications, counseling, and housing placements, implied that her life had become increasingly more dangerous and life-threatening until she was hospitalized in old age and protected from herself.

My son, Michael, entered a more enlightened treatment period, but I knew our family lacked the education and training to intervene adequately in time to protect him from severe psychotic episodes. Our first effort at outpatient intervention was largely fruitless, as the doctor conflated adolescent acting out with mental illness, offering only bland efforts to help our son. Failure to recognize Mike's problems, including extreme mood changes, inability to concentrate or learn, prolonged fears and anger, difficulties in sleeping habits, increased hunger, overuse of drugs and alcohol, and violent outbursts—all proved detrimental to Mike's recovery and dragged his mental illness into a protracted state. I am convinced that the initial holdup into in-patient treatment unnecessarily delayed Mike from essential treatment for his psychosis.

Sharon's and Mike's enduring and severe mental illness have been exacerbated by the glaring stigma involving family and patient blaming and hiding the problem. It is not only families but also the inadequate mental health support that seeks to minimize, ignore, or punish the sufferer who forgets to take medication, acts out in public areas, or violates the strict public housing codes. For the homeless mentally ill, not complying with city codes when living outdoors can earn jail time, which is hardly the setting of choice for a deranged person.

Like other mothers, I have experienced shame and self-blame for my son's mental illness, a condition that one woman describes as "bleeding inside" (Smith, 2022). I know Mike's father experienced similar troubled feelings, but he rarely confided to anyone about them. Lessening the stigma will indeed reduce this harmful condition.

The multi-generational nature of mental illness has been a rugged cross to bear. Among my descendants, four of my six children have lived with addictions, all but two of whom are now clean and sober—five of the ten grandchildren struggle with mental disorders or addiction. With five great-grandchildren, one is diagnosed autistic, and the other is psychologically unstable at 13. But we are no longer in the dark ages. Parental awareness, training, therapy, twelve-step programs, medication, and spirituality work wonders. All of these loved ones can expect to live full lives if they stay aware and sober.

Compassion, not criminalization, an updated model for intervention, offers a vibrant array of therapies, including ways to avoid long-term hospitalization. Community mental health should be precisely that: community-based. Our society must treat the mentally ill where they live instead of imposing one hospital regime after another that only temporarily halts the disease but fails to conquer it. The lack of available community mental health means too many patients cycle through psychiatric hospitals and are dispatched into the community while still unstable. Without a coherent community mental health system for the patient's immediate and long-term follow-up, including social resources of job, housing, nutritional food, and a friendly counselor who understands their situation, hospital time is simply an interlude, not a solution.

The National Alliance on Mental Illness summarizes the different types of therapy for bipolar disorders our family did *not* have available, at least at the beginning of Mike's psychiatric breakdowns. Variants of these therapies can also be helpful for other mental or emotional conditions. The trick is to develop the political will to finance mental health, educate the public, and provide the services required for this disadvantaged population.

My son is not alone in coping with serious mental illness. An estimated seven million adults in the United States have a bipolar condition, causing dramatic shifts in mood, energy, and cognition. Among these, 83 percent suffer severe impairment. Bipolar disorder is heavily stigmatized, leading to public misinformation about the disease (Ponte, 2022). As most of the therapies under discussion show, intensive interaction between the patient and care provider is required.

Family Focused Therapy (FFT). This therapy involves the family, spouse, or other family members. FFT typically lasts about 12 sessions (depending on the family's needs) and is provided by a single therapist. The focus is education: symptoms and how they cycle over time, their causes, recognizing the early sign of new episodes, and what to do as a patient and family to prevent the episodes from worsening. Later sessions focus on communication and problem-solving skills to address family conflicts.

Studies show that FFT and medication after an episode result in the patient having less severe mood symptoms and better functioning over a one-to-two-year period than those who get medications or case management. Admittedly, our family sessions attempted some of this, but the psychiatrist never educated Mike or us, his parents, to identify his symptoms or to let the family know when his cycling was speeding up. Mike spoke a few times about his rapid cycles and inability to control his mania. Still, I lacked the understanding to know how profoundly this affected him.

Interpersonal and Social Rhythm Therapy. This approach is individualized therapy in which the bipolar patient keeps daily records of bedtimes, wake times, activities, and the effects of changes in routines on their moods. Challenging problems—getting along with others, maintaining relationships, or other conflicts—can be discussed, and solutions offered. Generally, when Mike's mood is down, he seeks solutions: call someone, play music, take a walk, and so on. Journal writing has been crucial for stabilizing his moods, a strategy Mike used well with one important exception: when he relapses into drugs or alcohol.

Cognitive Behavioral Therapy (CBT). This individualized therapy focuses on the relationship between a person's thoughts, feelings, and behaviors. The patient learns to identify negative assumptions and thinking patterns and to challenge themselves to rehearse more adaptive ways of thinking. Another tool is to monitor activity levels to ensure they are engaged with rewarding aspects of their environment when depressed and are not overly stretched when manic. When Mike is stable, he remains sensitive to his negative thoughts and feelings and has acknowledged from time to time that he needs to "calm down" or "get positive."

Dialectical Behavior Therapy (DBT). A skills-based approach, this therapy teaches mindfulness and acceptance skills, such as the ability to experience moment-by-moment thoughts, emotions, and their accompanying psychical sensations without negative judgment. It also teaches distress tolerance, emotion regulation, and interpersonal effectiveness. I am uncertain whether Mike has had specific training in this therapy, but his periodic inability to link his thoughts, emotions, and physical symptoms suggests this strategy is missing in his toolbox.

Group Psychoeducation. Rather than a bipolar group get-together, Mike tells me over and over he has chosen the twelve-step program to reduce his feelings of isolation. Telling one's story and getting support and suggestions from others who have experienced the same situation has been highly beneficial for many. This tool has worked for Mike when he attends—but he attends only rarely. The significant problem is that Mike believes he no longer needs the Twelve-Step assistance.

Ruptures in therapy can derail any mentally ill person. The critical point is the continuity of individual or group therapy with someone who knows a person well, makes them feel comfortable, and encourages them to disclose essential issues. Medications and support from mental health professionals, who understand the journey, are crucial to an effective treatment plan and recovery.

Mike's treatment program once included a trained assistant who visited his home, helped with household tasks, bought groceries, or hung out with him. This support stabilized Michael and gave him a sense of having ongoing assistance. But once they pulled these supports away—claiming Mike no longer needed them, their misreading of his diagnosis—Mike lapsed once again into psychosis.

I recently encountered the term "anosognosia," describing a symptom experienced by those with serious mental illness. This warning sign occurs when a person cannot recognize their mental illness, which prevents meaningful communication about intervention or anything else that impacts the disturbed person's life (Lockard, 2022). Mike has frequently experienced this condition over the years and appears trapped and unreachable for real interaction during these episodes. For this mother, it has been heartbreaking.

But I remain hopeful that Mike has a wondrous encounter with Universal Love and joins the dance of Divine Mercy all around him.

Spirituality, often left off the list of therapies, actually plays a highly significant role in recovery. Living life meaningfully, avoiding negative self-judgments, and perceiving oneself as part of a larger whole of humanity helps surmount fear and defeat. Surrendering oneself to a Higher Power (whatever that means for the individual) takes the emphasis off the limited ego to embrace the larger picture. Although I've urged Mike to embrace organized religion, he tells me he's more comfortable with his personal spiritual program. Connecting with the stars on clear nights has been remarkably healing for him over the years. I pray he may allow the stars to guide him to sanity and well-being again.

A summary of therapies for the reader to take away:

Recovery as a Lifelong Process

Accepting Help

Caring for Self

Cognitive Rehabilitation

Spiritual Practice

A final note from the Buffalo Colts Football Team, who are supporting a mentally ill player, speaks a need for all of us: "Kill the Stigma!"

BIBLIOGRAPHY

Mental Illness and Substance Abuse

A Gentle Path Through the Twelve Steps: The Classic Guide for All People in the Process of Recovery, 7th Edition by Patrick Carnes, Ph.D., Center City, MN: Hazelton Publisher, 2012.

Anosognosia: A Big Word for a Surprising Condition by Trish Lockard. NAMI: National Alliance on Mental Illness. https://nami.org/Blogs/NAMI-Blog/August-2022/Anosognosia-A-Big-Word-for-a-Surprising-Condition

Bipolar Disorder Explained by Frederick Earlstein. Amazon.com, Pack & Post Plus, LLC, 2014.

Dual Diagnosis: A Treatment Approach to Mental Health and Substance Abuse Issues. Dr. Michael A. Gray. Create Space, 2018. Paperback.

Shifting the Research Lens: Mothers of Adult Children with SMI by Judith Smith. NAMI: National Alliance on Mental Illness. https://nami.org/Blogs/NAMI-Blog/August-2022/Shifting-the-Research-Lens-Mothers-of-Adult-Children-with-SMI

The Neuroscience of Addiction, Cambridge Fundamentals of Neuroscience in Psychology. Cambridge, England: University of Cambridge, 2018.

The New York Times, "It's Not Just You: America's Mental Health Crisis Isn't Just About Feelings. It's about Money, Power, and Politics, Too." October 16, 2022.

Understanding Bipolar Disorder by Katherine Ponte, JD, MBA, CPCR. NAMI: National Alliance on Mental Illness. https://nami.org/Blogs/NAMI-Blog/August-2022/Understanding-Bipolar-Disorder

Understanding Mental Disorders: Your Guide to DSM-5 by American Psychiatric Association. Washington, D.C.: American Psychiatric Publishing, 2015.

Personal and Inspirational Stories of Caregiving

Breathing Underwater: Spirituality and the Twelve Steps by Richard Rohr and Anne Lamont. Albuquerque, NM: Franciscan Medium, 1989; 2011, Paperback.

Care for the Caregiver: Surviving the Emotional Roller Coaster by Sherry Blake. Atlanta, GA: Dr. Sherry Enterprises, Inc., 2020.

Caregiving Our Loved One: Stories & Strategies That Will Change Your Life by Nanette J. Davis. Bellingham, WA: A House of Harmony Publication, 2012.

National Alliance For Mental Illness (NAMI). Advocacy and Educational Group. http://www,namiwa.org, Email: info@nami.org.

The ABCs of Caregiving: Words to Inspire You by Nanette J. Davis. Bellingham WA: A House of Harmony Publication, 2013.

The ABCs of Caregiving: Part 2, Essential Information for You and Your Family by Nanette J. Davis. Bellingham, WA: A House of Harmony Publication, 2015.

The Mindful Caregiver: Finding Ease in the Caregiving Journey by Nancy L. Kriseman. Washington, D.C.: Rowman & Littlefield Publishers, 2015, Paperback.

The Unexpected Journey of Caring: The Transformation from Loved One to Caregiver by Donna Thomson and Zachary White. Lanham, MD: Rowman & Littlefield, 2019.